FROM HARVARD

TO HELL

. . . AND BACK

FROM HARVARD to HELL
...AND BACK

A DOCTOR'S JOURNEY THROUGH ADDICTION TO RECOVERY

Sylvester "Skip" Sviokla III
WITH KERRY ZUKUS

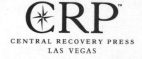
CENTRAL RECOVERY PRESS
LAS VEGAS

Central Recovery Press (CRP) is committed to publishing exceptional materials addressing addiction treatment, recovery, and behavioral healthcare topics, including original and quality books, audio/visual communications, and web-based new media. Through a diverse selection of titles, we seek to contribute a broad range of unique resources for professionals, recovering individuals and their families, and the general public.

For more information, visit www.centralrecoverypress.com.

Publisher: Central Recovery Press
             3321 N. Buffalo Drive
             Las Vegas, NV 89129

18 17 16 15 14 13   1 2 3 4 5

ISBN: 978-1-937612-29-0 (paper)
        978-1-937612-30-6 (e-book)

Publisher's Note: This is a memoir, a work based on fact recorded to the best of the author's memory. Central Recovery Press books represent the experiences and opinions of their authors only. Every effort has been made to ensure that events, institutions, and statistics presented in our books as facts are accurate and up-to-date. To protect their privacy, the names of some of the people and institutions in this book have been changed.

Cover design and interior layout by Sara Streifel, Think Creative Design

CONTENTS

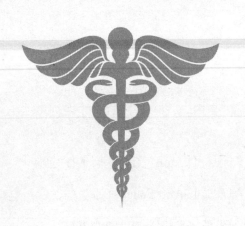

FOREWORD

Among United States adults, 12.5 percent report alcohol
dependence and 2.6 percent struggle with drug dependence during
their lives. That means that one out of every seven people in the
US has struggled with addiction at some time. Substance abuse
is clearly one of the most costly health problems in the country.
National estimates of the costs of illness for thirty-three diseases
and conditions ranked alcoholism second and drug disorders
seventh. The social costs of addiction are wide-ranging: medical
consequences, crime, lost earnings due to substance-abuse-
related illness and premature death, goods or services related to
crashes, fires, and criminal justice. In addition, a 2008 survey by
the Substance Abuse and Mental Health Services Administration
(SAMHSA) found that 11 percent of respondents with a substance-
abuse problem reported suicidal thoughts in the past year, and

2 percent made a suicide attempt in the past year (compared with 3 percent and 0.3 percent of respondents without a substance-use disorder, respectively).

Yet for all the information that supports that addiction is a serious, life-threatening illness, with arguably only moderately successful treatment approaches, most people are not appropriately outraged by this fact. Reasons for the lack of concern often stem from beliefs that people with addiction "do it to themselves," that people with addiction are of "low moral character" to begin with, and that this illness does not affect "people like us." These proffered reasons for the continuing stigmatization of addicts are difficult to understand in light of decades of scientific research on addiction. That is, until we consider that most people do not read arcane medical texts. Addicted individuals are relegated to either hiding their struggles or living lives as second-class citizens. If individuals with cancer were consigned to this same social dilemma, there would be an outcry. There is rarely an outcry for individuals with addiction.

I first met Dr. Sviokla (and I purposely use his title as he has definitely earned this sign of professional respect) when I was running a weekly group for physicians with substance addiction in Rhode Island. At that time he had been in recovery for a while, wanted to start a new life, and wanted to practice medicine again. Skip told the group about his background, his medical training and career, his descent into addiction, the effects of addiction on his family, and his hopes for the future. Even among a group of physicians who kid themselves that they are impervious to emotions, Skip's story was powerfully moving. Although the details of the story are gripping, the true impact of Skip's journey resides in his relentless hope and optimism to manage his illness and make his life meaningful.

Whenever someone comes forth to discuss his or her struggle with an illness, there is usually a huge response from people who have been suffering in silence. The first step in increasing recognition of addiction is to have someone like Skip humanize the illness. Stories such as Skip's—about brilliant, successful people struggling with addiction—are hardly rare, but they are rarely discussed in public. It is perhaps easier to think of the addicted individual as the homeless man who "chooses" to drink, who lies and steals and is therefore "not us." Skip's story demonstrates that addiction does not discriminate based on social class. In fact, he was both the homeless man on the street and the Harvard-educated doctor, athlete, father, and husband. He was the doctor who saved lives in the ER, who was engaging and brilliant, and who made others feel calm and safe and cared for. He was also the person who internally struggled with a life-threatening illness that for a period of time tore him and his family apart. His story, like any story of addiction, cannot be dismissed as "not like us." And that is perhaps what makes it so powerful and so disconcerting. Elite education, wealth, social standing, and a loving family do not protect us from addiction.

My patients with addiction often feel hopeless about their futures. I have always wished that I had a book like Skip's to give them. It's the story of a man who was able to face addiction head-on and overcome it. Skip is living proof that there is no reason stigma should be attached to this illness. It takes tremendous courage to admit to having addiction and to seek help. It also takes courage for someone to face his fears and to follow through with his treatment.

Dr. Sviokla has written a book for people with addiction, their families, and their friends and loved ones. It's a book we have all been waiting for—one that will entertain, inspire, and enlighten. As a physician working in this field, I know that denial, secrecy, and silence are the biggest barriers to treating addiction. I strongly hope that Skip's story will galvanize people who are struggling in silence to seek and receive appropriate help.

Jon E. Grant, JD, MD, MPH

Professor

Department of Psychiatry and
Behavioral Neuroscience

University of Chicago

Pritzker School of Medicine

ACKNOWLEDGMENTS

I offer amends to all those people I have not yet reached nor am likely to find. To Carole and Donald, for your teaching, example, and support I am truly grateful. To my children and grandchildren, my love and admiration for each of you floods my life daily. To Maurine with all my love, thank you for saving my life.

Because of these people and many more who have helped me, I am able to say this to those who still suffer: The journey back from hell can happen for you. I have learned that surrender does not merely cease hostilities in this war against substance abuse; it actually assures victory . . . and in this victory lies true joy.

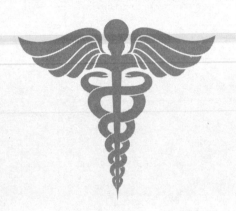

A LETTER FROM MY DAUGHTER

My dad is a father, a husband, a brother, a son, an uncle, a cousin, a teacher, a grandfather, a friend, a healer, a giver of life. There was no better place to be when I was young than the hospital. Usually a hospital is an overwhelming, sterile, scary place to be, usually a place to hope and wait for some sort of news. But for me, it was pure joy. My father walked those halls with a big white coat and a smile. He loved to show off his kids, and as a little girl I loved to show off my own hero, one who saved lives, healed hearts, and mended souls.

What I didn't know about my dad was that underneath his bigger-than-life personality there was a man who had his own set of demons, struggles he faced every day, struggles he never let any of us know about. His day consisted of making his family feel better and strangers' lives stronger, all the while ignoring his own pain. It's a pain I knew nothing about, a pain that was greater than he was. Ultimately, it was a pain that brought him to his knees. It was like waking up in the middle of a bad dream and begging for it to go away, but it never did. My hero had become a different person. It was like he had vanished. The big hands I loved to hold and chest I cried on over cuts, bruises, break-ups, and mistakes, had vanished. How could this man who always made you feel good about yourself feel so bad? I will never know how my father felt in those years of alcoholism and addiction. All I remember feeling in those years was fear. I feared every day and night that he would never come home, that we had lost the man who had made all our dreams come true.

And then he came back. Our father came back to us. He came back with no money, no pride, no job, just his big hands and trusting heart. He was ready to fight his demons. His sobriety amazes me. His path in life to heal other addicts, his need to give them their lives back, amazes me. I thank God every day my hero is back. This world is a better place with him in it. I wouldn't change any part of our past because all the challenges make my dad the dad he is, the dad he was, and the dad he always will be—mine.

From Amanda, Father's Day, 2009

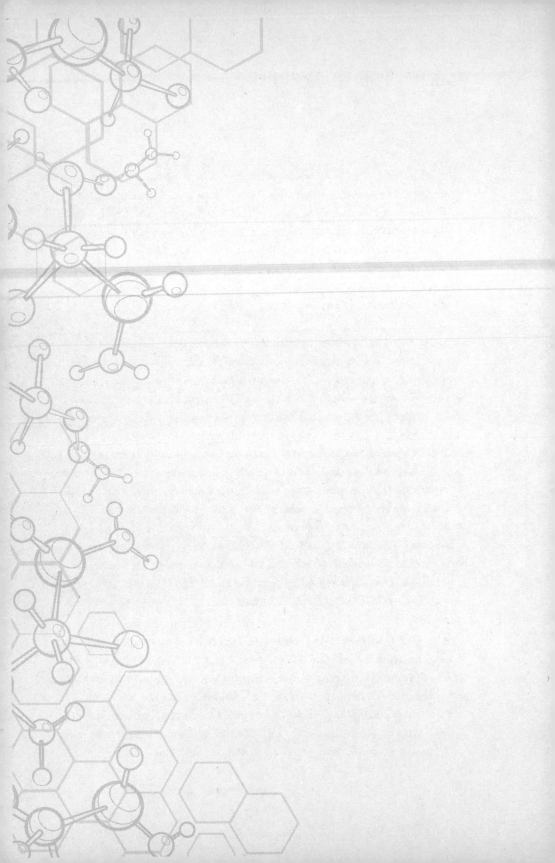

CHAPTER ONE

PILLS ON THE FLOOR

As I opened the pill bottle with great anticipation, one Vicodin lost its way and landed on the floor, skipping and sliding away to parts unknown. Since I took one hundred and fifty of these little babies each day, what was one stray pill to me but a penny to a millionaire? Yet I immediately dropped to my knees, searching for it like a near-blind man feeling around for a precious contact lens. I didn't care who saw me or what I looked like. If I couldn't see or feel the pill, I would have licked the floor to try to grasp it with my tongue if I'd had to.

This should have been the bottom, the message from God or whomever that there was no lower for me to go. I was on my knees. How metaphorical. But I was too sick to notice or care. I would have to drop down many more rungs on my descent to hell before any of that would hit me. Right now, all I needed was that one pill. Every pill mattered.

Over the years I'd serviced the medical needs of some of the biggest rock stars in the world. I kept their secrets and confidences. Some of them were addicts, but I'd never allowed myself to be used to enable those habits. I stretched some rules now and then, but I never crossed that line. I was no pusher. The closest I ever came was when the lead singer of a 1970s super group needed a shot of Demerol right as she came off the stage, which was my idea, not hers. She had shingles, a broken foot, and was in incredible pain. She didn't ask for it specifically, but she was from the "show must go on" school of thought and I respected what she'd been trying to do. There were thousands of fans waiting to see her on the next date of her tour and she would not disappoint, even if it damn near crippled her. I injected her because she'd danced on that broken foot, as she would every night. But that wasn't addiction. Me, I was an addict. For myself, I would do anything. I had no ethics whatsoever.

Most people start opioid addiction—and Vicodin is an opioid in the same family as heroin—because of pain. It's a painkiller. Was I in pain? No. I had once been in pain, but that was a long time ago.

I had closed the three weight loss clinics I owned in Massachusetts, moved out west, and over time ballooned up to four hundred pounds. The irony was completely lost on me. Instead of incorporating the very methods I had profited from, I went the "easy" route: gastric bypass surgery. With all surgery there is the immediate aftercare regimen of painkillers. Everybody gets them. But not everyone is an addict.

People take painkillers to kill pain. Addicts take painkillers for different reasons. The normal mind says, "I'm still in pain. I believe I'll take another," or "I'm no longer in pain. I believe I'll stop." The addicted mind says, "How many are in the bottle?" For most people, taking Vicodin as prescribed does not make them high in any way. It simply dulls their pain. But take a fistful of them and the energy and euphoria begin. I was all for energy and euphoria.

It's odd it took me so long to get into opioids. As a doctor, I always had access to them. I had access to damn near everything. But I cycled through substances like someone who took up various hobbies over the years. Many times I had no manifestations of addictive behavior at all. I just liked to party now and then, and I would do or take whatever recreational alteration was being offered by the host or hostess. The next day I'd be back at work—no need to continue feeding the beast, so to speak. For this reason, I never regarded myself as an addict, which is usually how it starts with addicts.

A person can occasionally take opioids for recreational purposes. I know because I had done it. But now I was chasing loose pills all over the floor. This was far different.

The truly addictive behavior did not begin immediately after my surgery. I abused painkillers then, but not so much that I couldn't quit them after a while. The irony was I was actually in more pain than most post-op patients. I had developed an infection. These things can happen.

Eventually, I switched from Vicodin to an anti-inflammatory that was nonaddictive and did not get me high. But that wasn't addressing the infection, so I instructed a nurse to inject me with antibiotics. She missed with the needle and hit my sciatic nerve. Now I was in *real* pain. Karma was kicking my ass over the weight-loss surgery. The damage inflicted continues to this day.

The infection was now gone, but because of the needle to my sciatic the pain was in overdrive, so I started taking Orudis, another anti-inflammatory. It began to work. It did not get me high, so there was no temptation to take more than prescribed. It didn't mess me up and I was able to work like a normal person—alert and on my game.

My gig at the time was medical as well as entrepreneurial, which is where the big money is. I owned an emergency room contract with a local hospital. I made sure doctors were working that ER twenty-four/seven, and I was responsible for paying them from the money the hospital paid me. To make a few extra dollars, I worked a few shifts a month myself. I was one of those "country club doctors." I worked a few hours a week here and there, and the rest of my time was for play. Meanwhile, the money rolled in. I was living large.

The more money you make, the more insurance you should carry, especially if you're a family man. I went for a policy-ordered physical and came through fine. Drug-free. Sorta. I was clean insofar as anything illegal, but I had a ton of protein in my urine, which was endangering my kidneys. I conferred with some colleagues and the diagnosis was that it was from the constant use of the Orudis. It was working great for me, but for my overall health I had to get off of it.

Without my anti-inflammatory, I was in excruciating pain again. But pain is relative. If I were treating someone else, I might have just switched him or her to Tylenol or some other over-the-counter remedy. It would have taken the edge off the pain and the person could have functioned fine. Then I remembered the buzz I got when I was doubling and tripling my prescribed dosage of Vicodin. That was fun. Now I had an excuse to do that again. With my own prescription pad in hand, back onto Vicodin I went.

I wrote scripts—prescriptions—for myself. When you're a doctor, this is no big deal. But I wasn't stopping at the dose required just to relieve my pain. I was taking enough to get me high, no different from a man who drinks until he is drunk. For a lot of people, it takes a lot of Vicodin in order to get high. Furthermore, the more you take, the more often you take it, the more it takes in order to get high. A fistful of Vicodin gave me energy and euphoria, and when you're rich and bored, who doesn't want a bit of energy and euphoria to give life meaning?

One pill, two pills, three pills an hour. It sounded like a sideline cheer, the kind I used to hear when I was starring on the gridiron at Harvard, but it was a dosing regimen and the numbers kept on growing. In no time at all, I was taking them by the fistful. How was I supposed to keep up with the demand?

I started writing scripts for my nurses. They didn't know I was doing this, but when you have a prescription pad, you can do a lot of things. Unimaginable things.

I didn't bring the nurses in as co-conspirators at first. I'd call in scripts in their names at the local pharmacies, places that were familiar with me, and say I would be passing by in an hour and I would stop by and pick it up myself. What a swell boss I was!

Still, the volume I needed required a lot of maximum-sized prescriptions, and opioids are controlled substances. It wasn't like I was writing scripts for acne medicine. Luckily, I knew a lot of pharmacies and I had a lot of nurses. Pretty soon, even that method got exhausted. You can only write a script for so much for a single person within a month before attracting the attention of the pharmacists, who have an obligation to be on the lookout for such things. I started calling in scripts using the names of my patients and my friends. Again, these people had no idea. Some I hadn't seen in years. Didn't matter. They were names, and all I needed were names.

Then I ran out of names. I started making them up. I was getting so impaired from the Vicodin I could have called in pills for John Doe or Jane Smith, but I was trying to be as careful as a drugged-out doctor can be in such a situation.

The pharmacists began to look at me suspiciously. I was seeing them as often as they were seeing their mailman. I widened my area of influence. I started calling pharmacies that didn't know me. This was harder but still doable. I'd drive all over the damn place, putting lots of miles on my car, driving while high as a kite. No matter. I had money, time, an "MD" after my name, a license number, a prescription pad, and a habit that was eating me alive. I was in heaven *and* hell.

My habit built up until I needed two scripts a day, for the maximum number of pills allowable per patient. I was chugging down two months' worth every single day. The logistics of this whole thing became a major undertaking. I was like the classic crooked accountant, the one who transfers money from account to account to account in order to keep his fraud going and not get caught. This was hard work! And despite being a Harvard man, I wasn't necessarily used to hard work. I was used to cruising by on natural talent alone. Things had always come too easily to me.

I finally started bringing the nurses in on the deal. I'd send them out to pick up the scripts. My face was beginning to draw too much attention. I was spending most of my days in pharmacies. At first I'd simply ask the nurses to fetch scripts written out for friends, other patients, or "ghost patients." Some pharmacies also delivered. Eventually, I'd write the scripts out in the nurses' names. They obviously knew this was illegal, but since I was their boss and they honestly liked me, they didn't balk too much. When one did, I would make something up like, "I need it for a patient who needs more than the pharmacist will allow, but he's in incredible pain and I approve of the override." I'd say just about anything. I was smart and thought fast on my feet.

Eventually, I made my way up to 150 pills per day. How I stayed alive I'll never know. My liver should have been destroyed by the Vicodin. I was over fifty—not a young man. Other guys my age were already retiring or talking about retirement. Me? I couldn't retire. It would mean I'd have to cut back on my high cost of living, which included the high cost of these pills. Health insurance doesn't cover drug abuse on this level, and besides, I was using other people's names on the scripts. If I'd asked for those bills to be submitted to the patient's insurance company, I'd have been caught and arrested within days.

Shortly before going crazy with the Vicodin, I was also drinking more than I should have been. That may not sound outlandish, but I had just had my stomach stapled. Guys with stapled stomachs aren't supposed to drink, or certainly not drink much. One needs a regular stomach and a normal digestive system in order to properly digest alcohol.

Strangely enough, I still kept up my shifts at the ER and no one who worked with me ever thought I was impaired. I was wise enough to not go to the hospital with booze on my breath. Drunk was harder to mask than high, so I had to time everything just right. I showed up on time, did my thing, and—luckier than any other single thing—I never made an error of judgment when it came to patient care. I didn't kill anybody. I was only killing myself and my family, but I didn't know that yet.

I always thought I held my liquor well. Then again, doesn't every drunk think that? My drink was Stoli, rocks. Before the weight-loss surgery, I used to go down to my private beach club and knock back six or seven doubles and no one knew I'd had a drop. Only a few weeks after the surgery, despite being told to either not drink at all, or at most to have a modest half-glass of wine, I tried to hit the Stoli again. I was an ex-football player, a man's man. Nobody told *me* what to do! But I could only get to around three or four doubles before people brought to my attention that I was sleeping with my head in a dish of pretzels on the bar. I'd toddle off to take a leak behind a nearby bush, then get awakened by an embarrassed club employee, pulling me out of the shrubbery I'd fallen into when I passed out, covered in my own urine. One bit of sanity I maintained was I didn't mix alcohol with the Vicodin. That could have been fatal and I didn't want to die, at least not yet.

By the time I was up to 150 Vicodin a day, I was no longer getting high. "High" means feeling something good. What I felt was no longer good. What I was doing, what I knew I was doing, was simply staving off the massive pain of opioid withdrawal. That thought scared me to death.

As smart as I thought I was, though, I hadn't really outsmarted the authorities. One pharmacist, from a pharmacy right near the hospital where I worked, blew the whistle on me. I'd used him first and I'd used him the most. I'd gotten sloppy and made him suspicious, so he contacted the state medical board about my prescribing practices. Unbeknown to me, the board had been tracking my activities for six months.

People on drugs get paranoid. "Paranoia" is unrealistic thoughts that others are watching you, following you, plotting against you, etc. My problem was I wasn't paranoid enough. I came to learn that the state board was interviewing all the pharmacists in San Diego County about me. Seems they weren't going to just put the fear of God in me by confronting me as soon as suspicions arose. They wanted me dead to rights. Their plan was to make an example of me.

One day I was driving to my home in La Jolla, California, when I saw a car parked out front and a group of people outside speaking to my wife. It was just a hunch, but it didn't look like it was because I'd won the Publisher's Clearinghouse sweepstakes. As I drove by, my wife's eyes met mine and I knew; I just knew. I peeled out and drove to a hotel. En route, she called me on my cell and told me to head home, we had a problem. That only propelled me faster in the opposite direction. I was blotto at the time and only had a handful of pills left. That I was high, driving, and had illegally acquired pills on me should have been my main concern. But in the state I was in, all that meant was, "Holy cow, I'd better get some more. My supply might be drying up."

I checked into a hotel in La Jolla, the fanciest place in town, and hid there. I used my own credit card and my own name. I was hiding in plain sight. This was not some clever ploy on my part. I was simply too addle-brained to make better decisions.

I made a few calls and it became clear all my options for more pills had been pulled out from under me, so I went down to the hotel bar and drank. And drank. I would go back to my room, empty the minibar, and sleep a bit before going back down to the bar, a very public bar, to drink some more. This behavior lasted for five days.

The term "social drinker" means "light drinker" to most, but to me it meant I liked to drink and socialize—a lot. I enjoyed chatting up bartenders and getting big pours. I tipped like Sinatra. I introduced myself to strangers and told wonderful stories to anyone who would listen. I was a gregarious, happy drunk who never admitted he was drunk at all. But now as I went from my room to the bar and back again, I occasionally got a bottle and took it back to the room with me. It was important. The bar wasn't open twenty-four hours, and I was out of pills.

Again, I could not bring myself to think I'd hit rock bottom. Drinking alone in the darkness of my room only served to block my cognizance, when it should have achieved the opposite.

People ask if the pain would have come back if I'd stopped taking the painkillers, and if that was the reason I kept taking the pills. The answer is yes and no. Whatever lingering pain I had from the damage to my sciatic was marginal. The problem would be drug withdrawal. That was a bitch and a half.

As soon as your opioid receptors, which have been overprimed for days, weeks, or months, are empty and looking for more opioids, your eyes become dilated, you get diarrhea, you're hot, you're cold, your legs twitch, and you have malaise like you wouldn't believe. It's a mess. It lasts around seventy-two hours, but then you are left with absolute fatigue. Believe it or not, a lot of addicts, if they can score, go back on opioids simply to get out of bed. The drug begins to act almost like a stimulant, providing much needed energy.

Everyone who does drugs does not become an addict. Everyone who goes through a period of addictive activity with opioids does not necessarily experience true addiction. This is genomic. Certain people are genetically predisposed to addiction. Nonaddicts can go through the physical withdrawal and not have the total lethargy an addict experiences. It's the ones who feel that adrenaline rush when they dose again after they go through withdrawal who are the real addicts. That's one of the prime litmus tests.

The Hollywood image of the opium den, where Eastern music plays and everyone lies around in a semicomatose state while sucking on pipes, is misleading. Many addicts work at high-powered jobs wearing a suit and tie, slip into the executive washroom, snort, swallow, or inject—and then go right back to a board of directors meeting. They get *high*; they do not lie on the floor like roadkill. This was how I was.

I did not call my wife. I did not call my office. I did not call my children. I did nothing any responsible adult would do or should do. I drank and hid. How long did I think I could keep this up? I had no idea, but it didn't matter. I had to keep a buzz on and I had to avoid the inevitable.

My wife knew very little about this entire debacle. I hid my addiction from her as I did from everyone else. There was no big drug stash under my sock drawer or anything like that. I'd get a bottle of pills and I would chug them down like a frat house beer. There was no evidence for her to find. If she had known the full extent of it, she would have intervened, but I closed her off. Maurine and I had been together since I was in medical school. She was the most beautiful woman I had ever seen. But drugs had become my mistress. I spent no time with my wife. She was living the sad life of a wealthy Southern California widow, even though her husband was very much alive. She didn't matter to me now. Our four children were all grown up and out of the house.

A lot of this had been brewing for years. I was susceptible to boredom, which is common among addicts. I took her for granted. It wasn't right and she didn't deserve it, but the way I was wired was also responsible for the good things in our life. I was always hustling for the next big deal, which allowed us to live like royalty. But I did not nurture her, nor did I nurture a lot of my business ventures for long, which was why I bounced from thing to thing. But now it was all about the drugs. How could I spend quality time, or any time at all, with my wife if all that mattered was scoring more drugs, doing them—a solitary activity by and large—and then doing the same thing all over again, round the clock?

Toward the end, right before the walls began to close in, the social aspect of my drinking was augmented by renting hotel and motel rooms where I would simply hide from life and live in my stupor. I was becoming too much of a fixture at certain bars and clubs. I'd want to get high before or after hours. I couldn't get high at home because my wife was there and she'd try to engage me, which I wanted no part of. The mistress analogy was apt. While other guys were slipping off to these sorts of places with young ladies, I was slipping off alone with my pills.

In the hotel, I spent laughably little time thinking about the crisis I was obviously in. I lived hour to hour, obsessed with staying high. Nothing else mattered. There was no long-term thinking whatsoever.

Meanwhile, the men in dark suits searched high and low for me. They returned to my house numerous times. They called people I knew as they continued to build their case. They figured I had to be sleeping somewhere, and knowing the lifestyle to which I was accustomed, they doubted I was curled up on the beach, covered in seaweed and garbage.

Maurine and my kids looked for me, too, but I wasn't being cooperative. They called the hotel, which was one of my regular hotspots, and got the front desk to admit I was registered there.

When I wouldn't even cooperate with my immediate family, Maurine reached out to a psychiatrist I'd been seeing. She asked him to go to the hotel to try and talk me into coming home and surrendering voluntarily to the authorities in order to bring this situation to some sort of resolution.

Getting this shrink to intervene was kind of a joke. I'd been lying to the man ever since I started seeing him. I was never honest in our sessions. He had no idea the extent of my drug abuse. But he found me at the bar, drinking everything they would serve me. Seeing him searching for me brought back the feelings of fear and depression I'd felt when I'd first driven past my house and saw the authorities there, which only made me want to drink more. I was in no shape to escape physically; I could only escape chemically.

The shrink did his patter and I must have freaked out on him enough that he went running out of the place. That's the most I can remember. I'm lucky I can remember any of this at all, and a lot of it comes from the recollections of others. In the sort of daze I was in, only certain visions, thoughts, and emotions remain. The idea that I would likely lose my medical license came and went. That was a biggie. It should have been bigger. It should have been the thing to kick me in the head and get me straight and ready to face the music, but that was too sober, mature, and logical for the state I was in. Instead, I kept drinking.

My wife kept calling me on my cell phone. Usually I ignored it, but she recalls me picking up once after the shrink ran out. She yelled at me and I deserved it. Through the fog, through the clatter, I got the message that my license was being summarily suspended, pending a hearing. In other words, due to their evidence in hand and my inability to be found, in absentia they canceled my ability to practice and write scripts. This would not be a long-distance, pain-free divorce from my occupation, though. I was still required to appear before them for a full hearing, along with possible criminal charges.

I had to get clean. I couldn't show up before these people stoned. That meant I also couldn't avoid the opioid and alcohol withdrawal forever.

I finally went home. There was the pain of the embarrassment; there was the pain of the withdrawal. I couldn't look Maurine in the eye. I spoke very little to her. I was sick as a dog and she took on the responsibility of explaining me away to the rest of the world. Meanwhile, I spent the next three or four days lying on the cold, hard bathroom floor, a complete wreck of a man. Pathetic.

When I finally got through the withdrawal, Maurine had already gotten me a lawyer. It was good one of us was straight enough to make adult decisions.

With the lawyer at my side, I finally surrendered myself to the powers that be. As we were going into the administrative building of the California Medical Board, he turned to me and said, "This is going to be a long walk." I thought he meant from our car to the office, but he was speaking in metaphor. It *was* a long walk. It was a walk from living as large as a man can to dropping to the bottom of the Grand Canyon.

They were rough on me. I was told to expect that, but still, I wasn't prepared for it. Being a doctor I was used to a certain level of decorum and respect. I got none. I was talked to like a common criminal. I *was* a common criminal; I just didn't have any grasp of it.

It was an inquisition. I'd been coached not to argue the facts. They had me dead to rights, so what was the point? When that's the situation, you're advised to throw yourself on the mercy of the court. They had no mercy for me. I was just the kind of guy they wanted to make an example of. Harvard college boy. Harvard Medical School. Big mansion in La Jolla. "Playboy" medicine—playing doctor to the stars, running fancy weight-loss clinics back east for people with unlimited money, playing the entrepreneur and working only a day or so a week yet making more in that week than most people make in three or four months. Yeah, I was the poster boy of "This is why I hate doctors." I was everything most people would like to knock off a pedestal.

They had copies of the prescriptions I'd written. They had testimonies of the pharmacists. They must have grilled the nurses something fierce because they gave me up, too. Some of those nurses also got in trouble, and I feel so bad about that. They asked if I ever gave any of the Vicodin to them, or if I ever shared it with anybody. I remembered myself crawling around on the floor so I wouldn't miss a single pill. Me, share? I'd have broken the arm of anyone who tried to grab any away from me.

I was tired of the running. This entire episode of my life had drained me. I was no longer getting anything good out of it. I was finished. I just wanted it to all be over so I could go on to the next chapter of my life, a chapter without the drugs and the subterfuge.

One of my inquisitors asked rhetorically, "How could you take all that Vicodin every day and still see patients?"

Before my lawyer could slap his hand across my mouth, I quipped, "I work a lot of night shifts, and most of the people who come into the hospital at that hour are real pains in the ass. A hundred fifty Vicodin makes them a lot easier to take."

That was not my finest moment. I recognized how they perceived me, which only made me want to play right into their stereotype. They thought I was an overprivileged asshole, so I acted like one. Bad idea.

Over the next few days my lawyer worked out the best deal he could. I was to surrender my medical license voluntarily. They would hold it, and if I could clean myself up during the next two years, they would allow me to reapply for my license and get it back. In the meantime, I could see no patients. As a doctor, I was done.

Like a cocky tough-guy criminal, I acted like twenty-four months would be a walk in the park. I had absolutely no idea what I would do with my life or how I would make a living. But I was still the golden boy. Nothing could ever hurt me.

One of the ironies of hitting rock bottom is few people recognize it when it happens. By the time it finally occurs to them, they've actually been on the ground for a long, long time. You can argue that my rock bottom was when I was scurrying around on my hands and knees looking for pills. If that wasn't it, surely it was when I was holed up in a hotel, drunk all day and all night, trying to dull the pain and avoid the "*Federales*" I knew were nipping at my heels. Or maybe it was going through withdrawal in my house while my wife turned her head away from me, unable to stomach looking at the sick bastard I'd become. But if it wasn't any of those, it had to have been when they took away the thing that defined me—my medical license. And yet I walked out of that administrative building with my chin held high. I'd been punched, and hard, but I wouldn't give the world the satisfaction of knowing it.

Once you do that for awhile, you begin to believe your own bull. I still didn't get it. I still thought everything was jim-dandy, and good ol' Dr. Skip was going to skip and dance once more. Piece of cake. Life was good. Life would always be good. I was immortal.

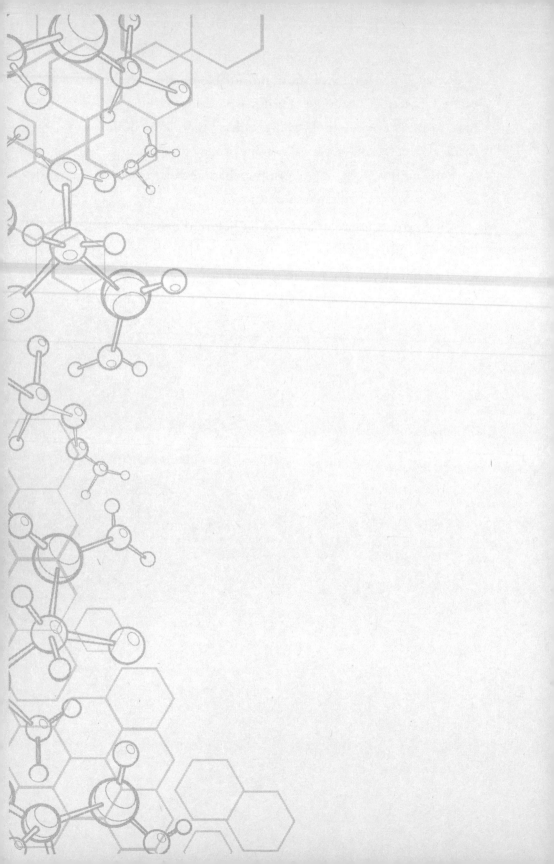

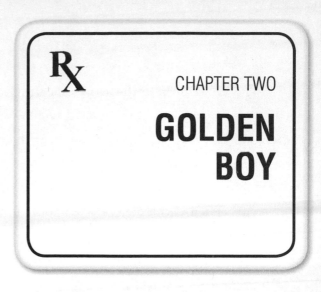

CHAPTER TWO

GOLDEN BOY

It would be easy and clichéd to claim my addiction was purely the result of my genetic makeup—that my mother or father or both were roaring drunks—but nothing could be further from the truth.

I was born and raised in Brockton, Massachusetts, the quintessential working class American industrial town. We were a microcosm of the early twentieth century: Immigrant groups coming in and settling down every few years, each a little wary of the others, each clustered together at first, fear driving wedges between each successive group until, working side-by-side, they were able to come to respect one another and create that classic melting pot that made us what we are as a nation today.

The Svioklas were Lithuanian. Upon arrival in Brockton, they settled in a section called the Village, which was where all the new immigrant groups initially set up shop. At the time my people came, the Village was mostly inhabited by Lithuanians and Poles. It was a ghetto in the classic sense, which does not mean it was crime-ridden and filled with ne'er-do-wells, but rather poor people who struggled to learn a new language and find their place in a new land before embarking upon their New World dream.

Brockton is famous for its shoe factories, and that sort of work was the most common starting point for the inhabitants of the Village, regardless of the skills and education they may have brought with them from their homeland. My father managed to avoid the factories, having been born in the US, so he was able to attend and finish high school in Brockton, doing quite well with his grades— so well, in fact, that he went on to Northeastern University in Boston, graduating with a degree in engineering. He was the first boy anyone could recall growing up in the Village and going on to graduate from college. Dad was a member of *Tau Beta Pi*, an honor society for the top 1 percent of the engineering graduates in the country. He was a miserably bright son of a bitch.

Everyone always talked about how smart Dad was, but my Scotch-Irish mother Katherine was actually the smartest person I ever met growing up—even smarter than Dad, although she never had the good fortune to graduate from college. They met at Northeastern, but when the war came he went into the Navy, while she dropped out and stayed behind, working as a draftsperson. My mother's intellectual brilliance made me a feminist as long ago as I can remember. She could have done anything and been the best at it. And strong women in my family did not begin and end with my mother. *Her* mother was incredibly literate. She lived with us and didn't die until she was 106 years old, and she had her own radio show at age 102. Along with that, she was a published author.

My grandmother's Scottish husband died young, falling off a skyscraper while at work, drunk. If there was any genetic link to addiction for me, that would have been it, but it was a slight one and rather far removed. I never knew the man, nor did I know how he died until I was well into my forties. On my Lithuanian side, drinking was verboten, even though there was a lot of drinking in the Village in general. Because of my Scottish grandfather there may indeed have been a bit of genetic predisposition for addiction, but certainly not an environmental one.

My father's father, "Sylvester the First," married his Polish sweetheart on the boat coming over from the old country. He immediately went to work in the shoe factories, working two shifts a day in order to save some money and get ahead. As soon as he had a few bucks he rented a second-floor flat, which he converted into a vegetable market. Soon he began extending credit to his Lithuanian customers, which eventually morphed into his loaning money outright. Today one might call him a microlender. Even after he started the store, he continued to work at the factory, and his wife put in a shift a day there as well. Finally, he was able to buy a building, where he installed a full-fledged grocery store on the ground floor. In the middle was a coal stove. He also had a real cash register that, when I was old enough, he allowed me to use, selling penny candy to my pals like a big shot. I loved that market. Every time I went there to see my granddad, I'd ask him what I could do to help. He always had something, although looking back, some of it was purely make-work work, like burying rocks in the backyard. Still, it instilled in me a work ethic, which was entirely the point.

All together, his ventures soon helped him become one of the more successful men in the Village. He eventually bought a few triple-decker buildings and rented them out. When my mother became pregnant with me, my family moved into the first floor of one of them, and Granddad and my father rigged the place with steam heat, which was a big deal back then, as the upper floors were all cold-water flats. From there, he bought buildings in Boston— about eighty or ninety apartments at his entrepreneurial zenith. When I wasn't tending store, I would go with my father to Boston to collect rent door-to-door. My father was a harder man than my grandfather. Dad would argue that we should evict people who got behind on their rent, while my granddad would say, "They're good people. They'll get back on their feet and pay us when they can."

I went to parochial school in Brockton. I was always large for my age, but Sylvester is not a great name for a kid, so I got teased and bullied a lot. It also didn't help that I was the classic "smart kid." Always with his hand raised, always quick with the correct answer in every class. Just the kind of kid you'd love to smack around to bring him down a few pegs.

My mother used to sing a little ditty that included the line, "You gotta be a football hero to get along with the beautiful girls." When I'd cry to her about the way I was getting bullied, she sang me that line and it began to sink in. Even at a very young age, beautiful girls were all over my radar. I vowed to myself that the first chance I got, I'd try out for a football team, learn the game, and find me some of those beautiful girls.

My father's brother was a Roman Catholic priest in Boston. I wasn't completely enamored of him. I thought he was a big blowhard—the "big" part because he stood six foot four with a muscular frame. He also drank a bit much, which made him the second person I was related to who abused alcohol, and although he had little direct influence on me, here again was a possible genetic link.

One day my uncle brought me into the kitchen of our home and said, "Skip, how would you like to go to the best high school in the world?" What overachieving eighth grader wouldn't be tickled to hear that offer? For whatever reason, I thought this meant going to school in England. It must have been all those old movies like *Goodbye, Mr. Chips*, with British schoolboys in their academic gowns. "I can get you into Boston College High School," he said. Getting me in was one brag; saying it was the best in the world was another, but this was his MO. I didn't know enough at the time to challenge him on BCHS being the best high school in Boston, let alone the world, considering Boston Latin usually held that honor. But Boston Latin was a secular school, and my uncle the priest wouldn't even put a secular school into the discussion.

My first two years I got a ride into Boston with a fellow from the neighborhood who worked around there. My last two years I'd ride buses and subways. Either way, it was a long trek, but I was attending "the best high school in the world," so I commuted proudly. Honestly, I did enjoy the school, and I found the Jesuits very academically strict, which was to my liking. I took Greek, I took Latin, and I loved it all.

When they announced tryouts for the freshman football team, I was the first man on the field, bright-eyed and eager. They took

one look at me and put me on the junior varsity. This had absolutely
nothing to do with my talent, which was nonexistent at the time. I
was just the biggest kid on the field and they figured they could put
me to good use somehow.

We played our games in the Fens, in Boston's Back Bay. My
mother would collect milk bottles for pocket change in order to
gather together enough money to pay her way on a bus to see me
play. My father could have easily afforded to give her the money,
but he was a tight son of a bitch and wouldn't do it, nor would he
let her drive. As much as I respected the hell out of my mother, the
chauvinist in the family was my dad, who should have looked at
her more as his equal. But she loved me and she would never miss
any of my games, despite having severe cardiac illness, worsened by
my father continually impregnating her against her doctor's wishes.
She died far too young and I always resented him for helping bring
about her demise.

At first I hardly played at all, as I was still learning the game and
my body wouldn't always do what my coaches and I wanted it to.
I can recall my mother coming up to me right after a particularly
abysmal game and saying, "I'm so proud of you. You have the
cleanest pants on the field!" To this day, I remember her acerbic
wit fondly.

I worked hard, got better, started the varsity as a sophomore,
and eventually made the all-city team and some all-state teams. BC
High also had a great boxing coach and I got interested in that as
well. Believe me, no one picked on me anymore. Academically I did
very well. Upon graduation, I received a first-place award in Greek
and in Latin, as well as a second in math. For as much as this was
supposed to be "the greatest high school in the world," I found it

easy. Mom was smart, Dad was smart, and I suppose I inherited a lot of their intellect.

Because of my rare combination of classroom smarts and athletic prowess, by my junior year I was being heavily recruited to play football by the top eastern academic schools, including most of the Ivies. Brown and Dartmouth were particularly intrigued and had me on campus for long weekend visits, which would soon devolve into typical frat house–type debauchery—quite an eye-opener for a young high school kid. Ladies and beer; ladies and beer. My, oh my, oh my.

Technically, the Ivies don't give out athletic scholarships, but back in the sixties they still managed to have certain academic scholarships that somehow seemed to always go to student athletes. Besides that, there was always need-based financial aid, a rather inexact science where again, recruited athletes somehow managed to get better deals than nonathletes from families of similar incomes. In short, it may not have been the kind of craziness associated with Division I schools like Notre Dame, Ohio State, and Florida, but there was still a lot of wooing and rule-bending in order to get decent teams on the field.

Boston College and Holy Cross weren't Ivies, but they both had stellar academic reputations, played ball at a high level, and liked me very much. Furthermore, both were Catholic schools, but once you've gotten bites from the Ivies, it's hard to look anywhere else. Perhaps if I were a top national recruit being flown around to USC and Alabama, my head might have been turned, but I was more of a regional recruit with top grades, so the Ivies were for me.

The local Ivy was Harvard, but more than that Harvard was . . . Harvard. Few are called and most answer. Harvard wooed me too, albeit in typical Harvard fashion. I spent a weekend there and the first thing the head coach said to me was, "You need to lose some baby fat." Everyone else was kissing my ass, but Harvard, as befitted them, kicked it. In its own strange way, that sealed the deal for me. The day college decisions came in the mail and my acceptance to Harvard was official, I sent them my deposit.

Despite that, Dartmouth would not be denied. I'd been there three previous times, but their coach asked me to come up once more to see if he could change my mind. He sent a private plane to get me and the wooing went off the charts. It was tempting but still, there's nothing like Harvard. I held to my commitment.

Outside of the beer parties on those recruiting trips, I drank very little in high school—maybe half a dozen times at most. Drugs of any sort were completely foreign to me. Some other kids drank more—and more often, but I had fallen into this role as the straight-A football star, prepping for Harvard. It was a costume I wore well.

In college things changed, as they do for most young people. The exhilaration of freedom and living on one's own leads college kids to sex, drugs, and rock 'n' roll, although for me it was more like sex, blackberry brandy, and rock 'n' roll. I saw drugs now—primarily marijuana—but for my first few years I stayed away from the stuff. I took football seriously, which dictated my partying behavior. If not for that, who knows?

By the sixties, Harvard and the other Ivies began moving away from their aristocratic ways. More kids like me—working-class kids from places like Brockton—were getting in on merit, rather than having their slots filled with C-students with names like Huffington Pufferton IV. Still, there were a few of those around and it felt strange to be rubbing shoulders with them. The Svioklas were living the American dream, but remained a few generations behind those cats with their Mayflower money.

I was more blown away by the academic prowess of some of the fellows I met, rather than the pedigrees of certain others. One of my roommates had seven perfect scores on his various SATs. I thought I was a big shot because I had one. But that's what Harvard is about—being intellectually humbled by your peers. Almost every kid there comes in with an oversized ego, the best his town ever saw. Then he meets his classmates and finds future Nobel Prize laureates and US Senators sitting next to him at the library, gobbling down knowledge like jellybeans at Easter.

I would not have traded my Harvard experience for anything else in the world. It was a wonderland of knowledge and I lapped it up like a hungry dog. Sure, some other guys may have studied more and attended classes more often, but the intellectual thrill was not limited to the classroom—it was everywhere you looked. At Harvard, you could take a seat in a dining hall and have all the academic stimulation you could ever desire. Every coffee house and doughnut shop in Harvard Square was a poet's corner. I was intoxicated, but in the best of ways.

Academically, I was all over the place my first few years, which, in my opinion, is as it should be. I tried this, I tried that, and I loved most all of it. In my first few years, I daydreamed of being an English major, eventually lying under the elms at some place like Oxford, reading the great masters.

I thought about medicine primarily because of my mother. Mom didn't push me to become a doctor. She was in poor health and I wanted to be the guy to save her. When I was in fourth or fifth grade, my father dropped my mother off at Mt. Auburn Hospital for heart problems she was experiencing following one of her many miscarriages. When he returned, he brought me into the kitchen and said, "Your mother's having heart surgery tomorrow and she might die." I knew she was sick; I knew she went to the hospital from time to time, but no one ever told me she was dying. That night I did not sleep a wink. By virtue of the work of a brilliant heart surgeon, my mother survived. But years later, my own path into medicine was still not set in stone.

I did well academically at Harvard—not that I worked as hard as some of the "grinds" or "tools," as the kids who practically lived in the library were called, but because I learned fast how to *get* good grades. Good grades are an art unto themselves. One must never confuse grades with knowledge, although I learned an awful lot in spite of myself. But I had yet to really be challenged.

College is also the time for kids to become political. Here, I stood out for really running against the grain. It was the sixties, in Cambridge, Massachusetts, and my politics could best be described as conservative-libertarian. My family voted for Kennedy because we were Catholic, but outside of that, my politics could not be further from JFK's.

Organizations like SDS, SNCC, and CORE were just starting up, as opposition to the burgeoning war in Viet Nam took hold, beginning primarily at the top universities in the land. My organic chemistry teacher was the guy who invented napalm, a defoliant he never intended to see used by the military. People would picket the poor guy's classroom every day and it pissed me off something fierce. I felt I had gotten to know him on a personal level and I knew he had no desire to see such a thing used against people or to make American soldiers sick. Experiences like that can color a person's entire political outlook.

Another fellow and I formed and comprised the entire membership of the Harvard Young Republicans. That's how outnumbered we were. We took turns being president. When Barry Goldwater came to Fenway Park during the 1964 presidential campaign, I carried a homemade sign in his support. I got peppered with so much fruit and vegetables I could have been a greengrocer. I was lucky to get back to my dorm alive.

Football was as humbling as academics. Even though it was an Ivy team, 110 guys showed up on the first day of practice and about ninety of them were all-staters. I thought I was at the University of Oklahoma or something! I expected a field full of little nerds and I'd be the big guy. Not so.

Back then, freshman couldn't suit up for varsity, so I played on the freshman team. I played a lot, although they tended to spread the minutes around pretty evenly to see what everyone was capable of, playing for the first time at a higher level. Still, I was pleased with my overall performance and once the season was over I couldn't wait for it to start up again the following year.

At Harvard, freshmen students all reside together in Harvard Yard. By sophomore year you are assigned a "house," a sort of residential college á la the great British schools like Cambridge and Oxford. I was slotted for Adams House. It was a lovely place, but I soon realized I was the only varsity athlete there. Talk about the differences between the Ivy League and most other colleges! No "jock dorms" for us. Although I befriended guys who had all sorts of interests, I felt secluded. It also put a lot of pressure on me when it came to intra-house athletics, where each house was expected to field a contingent and fight for the honor of the house. I'd been stuck with all the little guys!

Sophomore year I played varsity as well as junior varsity (JV) football. On JV, I played a ton of minutes, playing on both sides of the ball as an end. I played some varsity, but not enough to letter, much to my disappointment. A handful of other sophomores did letter and that got under my skin. I was good but I must have been doing something wrong, yet I couldn't figure out what it was.

Like a mindreader, one of the assistant coaches came up to me and said, "Skip, you're playing out of position. You really ought to be a defensive tackle." Bingo, a light went on. I spent the off-season lifting weights and getting myself into the proper body shape to excel at this new position.

It worked. I began preseason as a third-stringer, but by the time camp broke, I was a starting defensive tackle. I had a great season, too, my senior year, and I made some all-Ivy squads and other such honors. Opponents began double-teaming me, which didn't help my stats any but it helped the team, and that was the important thing. Cornell double-teamed me for an entire game and we beat them twenty-one to zero because they left the linebacker behind me unguarded and he made tackles all over the place. I was not only getting written up in *The Crimson* and other such Harvard publications, but also the the *Boston Globe* and the *Boston Herald*. Hell, I was parodied in the infamous *Harvard Lampoon*. That's when you *really* know you've made it. I even got one vote for the Heisman Trophy.

At the time, there was no NFL Scouting Combine as they have today, but they had the precursor to it called BLESTO-V, which was an acronym for Bears, Lions, Eagles, Steelers, Vikings

Talent Organization. These teams worked together organizing a tryout camp for NFL prospects. One team might invite you, but their partner teams also got to see you go through your paces. The Chicago Bears invited me and I thought I'd hit the lottery. Me, a kid from Brockton, a Harvard man, being asked to try out for the NFL. I harbored no delusions of NFL grandeur, though. I knew who I was and how I measured up. Those pros were on an entirely different level. I knew deep down inside my future lay in what my brain, not my body, could do. Still, I dreamed the strangest dream. I dreamed of going to camp with the Bears and having Dick Butkus knock my block off. They thought I was too small to play NFL defensive tackle and wanted to move me to linebacker, where I'd be competing with the legendary Butkus for a job. As if.

Ivy guys rarely made a dent in the NFL. Each senior year, as players strode off the field after The Game—the great Harvard–Yale rivalry and each team's last game of the season—we'd look up at the sky, win or lose, thinking to ourselves, "It's over. Football is over for me. Ah, I'm going to miss it." I saw my old teammate, Oscar winner Tommy Lee Jones, verbalizing that very sentiment on TV not that long ago. I enjoyed a locker room friendship with that soft-spoken tough guy from Texas, who took kidding about his love of the theater in good stride. *And he was a very good player!* But that's the sort of people you'd meet playing at Harvard—no dumb jocks but Renaissance men who just happened to have an appreciation for the body as well as the mind.

Football defined me at Harvard, but after The Game, I knew I had to consider my future without it. After my brief flirtation with English, anthropology was perhaps my greatest pleasure, but when I'd talk to my dad about it, he'd say, "And what do you expect to do with that?" Truth was, the most common answer was teach, and teaching didn't really turn me on, nor did the prospect of graduating Harvard and looking forward to merely earning a teacher's salary for the rest of my life. Making lots of money and doing better than my dad and my granddad had been drilled into me from birth. A teacher's salary would have been a lateral move at best.

Back when I was a young kid, and my mother nearly died of heart disease, a great cardiac surgeon gave her many more years of life through his knowledge and ingenuity. I recalled so vividly when he came out in a brown tweed three-piece suit to inform my father and me that my mother had survived the ordeal. That image stuck with me, as it did my father. The man in the three-piece suit was a miracle man, the image of every ideal we, as a family, held dear— brains, hard work, accomplishment, prestige, wealth, and humanity. Sometimes it was said to me directly, sometimes not so directly, that this is the man I should aspire to be.

I took the bait. I made my major biology.

Once I decided to pursue medicine, I was advised to get some experience under my belt in order to impress on my med school applications. While still an undergrad, I wandered over to Massachusetts General Hospital, one of the best in the nation, willing to do just about anything.

It was there I came in contact with Dr. Howard Baden, a dermatologist by specialty, who was an amazing scientist doing major cancer research. The man was brilliant—he had graduated at the top of his class at Harvard Medical School, where I dreamed of being accepted. I took a job cleaning and organizing Dr. Baden's research lab. He took a liking to me and gave me more responsibility. This culminated in his allowing me to present his work to the National Cancer Institute as an undergrad. That was an honor. Although my name was on the paper, it was his work, yet the fact he included me spoke to his great generosity.

Dr. Baden and I were wired differently, that was for sure. He would tilt his head and look at me like I was a T-Rex walking on its hind legs. The man had no interest at all in sports, yet there I was, a young guy known only for his prowess on the football field, a place completely foreign to him. I'd try to tell him about my exploits and all he would say was, "Doesn't that hurt?" He was a practical fellow, and a collision sport like football was not, on many levels, very practical, especially to a practitioner of medicine. Yet I latched onto him, and he became my mentor.

There are many great medical schools in the world, but going to Harvard College plays on the brain. Suddenly no other place holds a mystique. I applied to Harvard Medical School and only Harvard Medical School. Foolish, I know. But I got in, which is all that counts.

Despite facing my imminent future as a medical student, I was still immature. I was having too much fun as an undergrad, especially once football was finally out of my life. It was football and my love for it and desire to succeed at it that kept me relatively on the straight and narrow throughout my undergrad years. My partying was mild and infrequent compared to most other students. Freed of that, I was like a newly released convict.

I wore a path to Wellesley to see all the pretty girls. I partied like a rookie, drinking to excess at times but not caring much about the consequences. Call it "senioritis," especially once I learned I'd sewn up a spot in grad school. I was introduced to pot, which was fun, but I was more enamored of the ladies than of drinking or smoking dope for its own sake. What I did with drugs and alcohol I did socially and nothing more.

If ever there was an apex to my life, I thought this was it. Football hero, Harvard man, ladies' man, party guy, about to enter Harvard Medical School and come out the other end with all the riches in the world to greet me. How could life get any better?

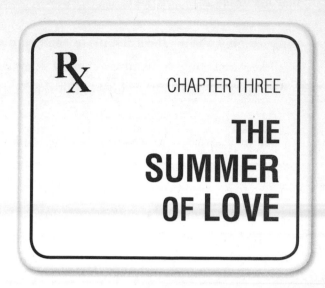

R̥x

CHAPTER THREE

THE SUMMER OF LOVE

Her name was Maurine.

In the summer of 1966 we met at her relatives' house on Cape Cod. I was on a date with another girl, but that didn't stop my wandering eye. Her cousin Paul and I were working together at Mass General and we double-dated a lot, which led to his magnanimous gesture of inviting me down to the Cape. Meeting Maurine was nothing more than an accident, but the moment I saw her I was smitten, yet couldn't let on for fear of being a cad. Still, I flirted as much as humanly possible, attempting to gauge her interest. This was made all the more challenging when the girl I was with kept dropping hints that she and I were bound for the altar even though I had said nothing of the sort and had given her little in the way of such encouragement.

Maurine was a slender blond with great legs she showed off in a purple miniskirt, and she had the most beautiful face I'd ever seen. I left Maurine with something vague like, "We ought to get together sometime," to which she seemed receptive. I knew how I meant it, but I had no idea if she was picking up on all my signals and hidden desires. Worse yet, she was about to embark on a year abroad at the Sorbonne in Paris.

As time passed, Maurine stuck in my mind despite our brief, chaste solitary day together. In the middle of the winter, though, I got a postcard from her from France. There was nothing earth-shattering in the message, but it was obvious she was trying to keep in contact. I think the two of us were feeling each other out, not wanting to be taken the wrong way, not wanting to express any interest when the other might be otherwise involved. But that postcard made my day. She remembered me. I had made an impression.

Once she came back from France it was another summer—1967, the so-called "Summer of Love." I had just graduated from college and was still in my "senioritis" mode, partying like a wild man, drunk on life itself—and whatever else I could get my hands on. The revelry turned up a few notches more once I knew I had gotten into Harvard Medical School and had a summer with no classes and no preparation for football. I was a free man with a few bucks in my pocket and the world by the tail.

I didn't waste any time calling Maurine and asking her out. From there things went great. I wasn't ready to commit right off the

bat, although I was thoroughly infatuated and we saw each other
often. Her cousin Paul and his mother, Maurine's favorite aunt,
must have thought the whole thing was a splendid pairing and did
everything in their power to push us along together. They'd invite
me down to the Cape often, which I'd have loved even if I had
never met Maurine. But it was clear they had matchmaking in mind.
Maurine's aunt would make a fantastic dinner and claim Maurine
had done all the cooking—only later would I learn she had not. But
it didn't matter. They might have thought I was a man in need of a
wife, but the concept couldn't have been further from my mind.

Medical school began in mid-August and I probably
anesthetized away some of my deep-seated anxieties about the place
through drinking. Underneath my cocky demeanor was an insecure
kid who knew he wasn't all that swift at math and science. Foolish
immaturity helped me get past those feelings when I'd first entered
Harvard College. Football made me a big man on campus in my
latter years. But now I was to be a struggling first-year again, and
this time I was worldly enough to know what I did not know and it
scared me. The partying continued.

First year of medical school is a lot of theoretical basics and I
found it challenging. But that year HMS tried something new—an
appropriately hippy-like concept of no grades. No grades! What
student wouldn't be thrilled by that? Grades meant competition, and
in the Summer of Love, competition sounded too much like war,
and war was bad.

Problem: grades are not just about competition. They are also
a way for a student to measure how he or she is doing. With no
grades, I bumbled and stumbled yet never knew how far I was
falling behind—or if I was behind at all. Grades are like pain. Any

doctor will tell you the most beneficial thing about pain is that it tells us something is wrong. I was a patient with no capacity to feel pain, so I thought I was well.

I wasn't.

Even tests went ungraded. From sixteen previous years of schooling I knew about grade curves and such, so even though I got tests back with red check marks on them, without a letter grade I couldn't grasp how badly I was doing. I knew I wasn't at the top of my class, but outside of that, I figured I was hanging in there and getting by. As the old saying goes, what do they call the guy who graduates last in his medical school class? "Doctor."

In Gross Anatomy, I was teamed with three women—three women and me on a cadaver. There were only about ten women (to about ninety men) in our entire class that year, so this was quite the oddity. As one might imagine, in dealing with the gender biases of that era, these women were incredibly accomplished. In lab one day I spotted a book entitled, *The Anatomy of the Guinea Pig* (scintillating reading I'm sure). Daydreaming, my eyes traveled to the name of the author. It was identical to that of one of my female classmates. Funny coincidence. The next time I saw her I made mention of it, simply as a way of making conversation. "That wouldn't happen to be a relative of yours, would it?"

"No, that's me. I wrote the book."

I was stupefied. "You wrote a textbook already? What the hell are you doing in my first year medical school class?" But that's what it took to be a woman in medicine back then—particularly one lucky enough to be chosen for Harvard Medical. My biggest claim to fame was getting a Heisman vote. Not quite as applicable to being a doctor.

The year 1967 was more than just the Summer of Love. If you lived in Boston, it was the year of the "Cardiac Kids"—the Boston Red Sox with Triple Crown-winning Carl Yastrzemski leading the way to the World Series. Every single game that year was a thriller, and as a sports fan, I just had to be there. Unfortunately, it seemed every daytime home game during the week took place on the day and time of my Gross Anatomy class. For a more mature person, this would have meant little. But I was immature. Plus, this was long before DVRs or smart phones or any of the other modern methods we have for watching games later or remotely. Also, there's nothing like being at the ballpark, and Fenway Park is a magical place, and 1967 the most magical of years. Grandstand tickets were only two bucks, and for a dollar or two more you could sit in even better seats, which I often did.

I cut class instead of cutting into a cadaver. Fenway was only a few blocks from school, so I could literally hear the games from campus—a siren's song. Weekday games also drew poorly despite how well the team was doing, so getting great seats was easy, making it all the more tempting.

My three lab partners were highly motivated and didn't seem to mind carrying my share of the load in my absence. Plus, since we weren't being graded as a group, it wasn't like my irresponsibility was harming any of them. I actually got the impression they were happy to have "The Neanderthal" out of the lab. Nice, hardworking, intelligent women covering me in class, and Yaz and Jim Lonborg exciting me on the field. Life seemed good.

I spent weekends with Maurine—as well as other girls—when I should have been studying. Wine, women, and sports dominated my life as they had in the summer, despite it now being fall. Gradually, I let the other girls pass from my life and spent more and more time with Maurine, who was matriculating at nearby Tufts University in Medford, Massachusetts. Maurine, meanwhile, was doing much the same, seeing other guys at first as well. We were both pretty up front about it all.

One day we were in an IHOP just outside of Boston. Maurine had met an Israeli guy while at the Sorbonne and he was coming into town to visit her. She told me all about it but by this point it did not sit well with me and I let her know it. "Goddamn it, you are not seeing that guy."

"Yes I am," she shouted back.

"No you aren't, 'cause you're going to marry me." This took her aback a hundred yards. After a long pause, she replied, "Are you asking me?"

"No, but either you're marrying me or I'm not going to see you again."

"Okay."

The whole thing came out of me with no forethought and afterward I almost wondered if I'd been tricked into it. Still, it was not an official marriage proposal, but I had made it clear to her how I felt. For the first time in my life I wanted an exclusive relationship and I wanted it with her. She didn't seem to mind.

Maurine was gorgeous, bright, multilingual; we had shared values and had the same ideas about family and children. Everything had already been coming into place, but now that I had said what I said— in anger and frustration, I might add—the entire picture started to take shape. *I think I'll marry this girl.* Yeah, that sounded like a plan.

Now I had another thing to occupy my busy brain. I wished I were about five years older and further along with my schooling and career, but I'd found the girl for me and I was afraid if I didn't make my move I might lose her. In a matter of weeks I doubled down and proposed to her officially—and not in a restaurant during an argument. She made me the happiest guy in the world when she said yes.

I went to my family and told them all about it. They were stoic rather than disapproving, asking all the logical questions: "How are you going to support her?"

"She graduates this spring and she's going to be a teacher. She'll get a job and work while I go to medical school." That seemed to placate my folks, although we all acknowledged we wouldn't be living like kings. But this scenario was typical, especially for our generation. Everyone wanted to marry a doctor, and if you did, you didn't mind supporting him for a few years while he became one. Better to nail one down before another girl snatched him up, although I had been the one trying to seal the deal with Maurine more than vice-versa.

My folks had no issues with marrying young, nor did Maurine's family. We set the wedding for June 15, right after the school year.

Meanwhile back at school, I staggered through. I felt some of the classes were easy while others were hard, pretty much as I'd felt all through my undergrad years. No problem. Harvard had a pretty good core curriculum so I wasn't coming in from some remote island of learning where everything was foreign to me. About a third of the class was from Harvard College and I figured we were all approaching things from a similar perspective. *All* the Harvard and Radcliffe people couldn't have been struggling, could they? I could only assuage my anxieties by ignoring them. We had no grades! It was frustrating, yet it also gave me an odd sense of calm. No pain—no injury. No grades—no failure.

Socially, I felt a bit isolated at school. I became kind of a loner. All the dorm rooms were singles and most everyone simply stayed in their room to sleep and study—no room parties or anything like that. People studied so much they were almost embarrassed about it, like they wanted others to think their fine performance in class was effortless. The guy living next door to me was such a nerd he even faked going away for spring break. He said he was going to Florida, but I came back early and saw an eerie glow under his door. I tapped and then knocked hard on his door. He sheepishly answered, trying to not let me notice the sun lamp he'd been using. He'd stayed on campus the entire break, catching up on his studies.

I had Maurine, but other than that, medical school is usually not as social as undergrad. They say law school and business school have a lot of study groups and such, but in med school you tend to be on your own. Perhaps if I'd been paired with some others I would have snapped to and pulled my own weight more, but instead I just drifted off. I had no football teammates to make me feel I was responsible for someone other than myself. Besides, if there ever were groups coming together to study I would have been the last guy asked. Early on I developed the reputation of being a "dumb jock," and instead of fighting it, I embraced it. Bad move.

Before I knew it my first year in medical school was coming to a close. I was certainly aware of what was going on around me, but Maurine, sports, and partying were at the center of my life far more than football had ever been, and certainly more than academia. I never really got out of the rut I'd claimed for myself once I finished my senior football season—too much nonsense in my head and not enough maturity. I began looking around me and feeling, regardless of grades, that I had to have been the least serious person in my class.

I wasn't some lost soul following the crowd off a cliff—I was *leading* that parade and didn't care whether anyone was following me or not. Still, the problem with failure is not always the inability to recognize it, but the unwillingness to do anything about it. I was in a hole—I knew not what its depth—and I just kept digging deeper.

My drinking increased. I dabbled in drugs, although not exactly recreationally. College and medical school students frequently play with speed and various forms of stimulants in order to keep awake and get work done. I'd goof off and then take some black beauties in order to get a paper done or be awake for a test. As for the drinking, the more I drank, the more I required in order to make the drinking seem worthwhile. I wouldn't say I had become an alcoholic by this point in my life, but I was on my way. I outdrank every other med student I knew. I justified that it was because I was so large and loomed over the rest of them. The human body is two thirds water. We're human drinking vessels. The other kids were shot glasses. I was a big ol' beer stein.

I may have done speed during the week but I kept most of my drinking to the weekend, so I convinced myself this proved I had no problem. All the other students drank on the weekend; why not me? And even though I outdrank them, I wasn't waking up in strange places without recollection, nor was I vomiting on people or wetting myself. No one ever asked me to leave a party because I'd gotten out of line. I'd get drunk, act a little silly, get tired, and then find a reasonable place to lay my head. Problem solved.

When the semester finished, I had only two days before my wedding. Needless to say, my mind was all over the place. The very day before my wedding, I got a phone call from the dean's office asking me to come over. I had no idea what was on his mind, but since I was about to be married and then off to a honeymoon, I figured it would be best to get right on over there and get it taken care of.

Sitting in his impressive office, the dean sat across from me and said, "I wanted to talk with you before you left. I'm sorry to be telling you this so late, and we should have notified you earlier, but you haven't been doing well."

This did not surprise me, but hearing it said to me so directly, and being called into the dean's office to hear about it made me feel all kinds of queasy. "How bad?"

"You really haven't performed well enough to move into the second year."

I was stone silent, in shock. Do that long enough and the other party will inevitably keep talking. He rephrased. "You haven't passed the first year."

Through a mouth as dry as sand I responded, "This is kinda shaking me up 'cause tomorrow I'm getting married."

"Well, why don't you get married. Are you going on a honeymoon?"

"Yes. Acapulco."

"Nice. Try to have a good time."

Easy for him to say.

". . . and when you get back, we have all agreed to test you and have you see a psychiatrist to figure out what happened and maybe we can help you work on your future."

All the prior shocks in my life had been pleasant ones—getting into Boston College High or getting into Harvard and Harvard Medical. These are the moments that make you go giddy and catch only the broadest essence of what is happening, causing you to go back moments later to revisit the details. In this case though, the news was the worst I'd ever been given—aside from being first told of my mother's failing health—and there was no ability to go back immediately and get more information. Was I out or was I still in? He'd made it crystal clear I did not pass. So why was I coming back for "testing"? And what did a psychiatrist have to do with anything? Did they think I was crazy? I *felt* crazy right about then. In less than twenty-four hours I would be wed. Now this.

I left the dean's office on wobbly knees. The scintilla of optimism that never leaves the body until the moment we die said, *But if it's all over, they wouldn't be asking me to come back after the honeymoon. There must be a chance I can rectify this. It must not all be over. All hope must not be lost.*

What happened next was a turning point in my life, yet I wouldn't grasp it until years later. I thought the news from the dean was a signpost in my life's road, but there was more. What would I *do* with this information? As a kid and a young man, up until this moment in my life I told about as many lies as your average person. I don't claim to be a saint. But those were little white lies. This was a major issue. Do I tell Maurine and my family or do I not?

I chose to lie. I told myself I would come clean to Maurine after the honeymoon. Meanwhile, I told lies of omission and commission. I lied like a rug. Your wedding is *your* day. Outside of your funeral—which none of us has the opportunity to appreciate—the day when you have all of the focus placed upon you by everyone you know is your wedding day. Every person there asked me about medical school. I lied. They asked about my future plans. I lied. Maurine lied on my behalf and she didn't even know she was doing it. Every single lie cut me like a knife because only I knew how wrong they were. But lies can give us calluses, in a way. The more we tell, the more comfortable we are telling them. By the end of my wedding day I was rolling with the punches. *Yeah I did great this year. Can't wait for next year. Yes, it feels great to be on the road to being a doctor. Maurine's going to provide for me while I study and then when I become a doctor, I'll bathe her in diamonds and pearls. Ours will be a great life. Thank you all for coming.*

I was a prodigious liar. And no lies were worse than the ones I told my new wife and my mother and father. I went through my entire honeymoon without saying a word about my situation to Maurine. Physically, the honeymoon was great, and the tropics were wonderful. Still, this Sword of Damocles hung over my head, taking some of the pure joy out of what should have been the most joyous week of my life.

On the plane home all I could think of was how I would break the news. It couldn't be avoided forever. We got ourselves a small apartment near the school and moved in as we'd planned, both of us acting like everything was hunky dory. One day I told her I had to go over to the school to do some research. Ha! Research. I was researching how to stay *in* the damn school! The dean promised me a meeting and now I went to have it, my mind filled with dread and anxiety.

The whole scene was odd. It was as if the administration were trying hard to provide me with excuses for my poor performance. This made no sense to me—and it still doesn't—but at the time it seemed like a lifeline being tossed to a drowning man. Maybe they didn't want to have a high dropout rate. Maybe if they had to fail kids they preferred they weren't Harvard College kids. I don't know.

They arrived at the conclusion that I did not know how to study. This was balderdash, but hey, if they wanted to make excuses for me, it was fine by me. How could a Harvard man not know how to study? I knew how to study; I simply chose *not* to study. I had chosen to goof off.

They spent three or four days giving me psychological testing for hours and hours. They had me put together puzzles and stick round balls in round holes. It was the sort of thing you have a monkey or a mentally incapacitated person do. This was Harvard Medical School? What were they testing me for, brain damage? But I went along. What other choice did I have?

Ironically, I'm not very good at those types of tests. I'm not wired for engineering, so when they had me using my hands to take puzzle pieces and make them into something of their choosing, I fumbled a lot. Orthopedics would never be my specialty. I'd get frustrated and mutter under my breath. The person viewing me made notes while I struggled, then stepped away for a moment, leaving her notepad behind. Maybe that was a test, too, and if so, I probably failed because I quickly grabbed it and read it. "Subject gets foul when he can't finish tasks in time." No shit.

Ten days went by, which felt like forever. I'd still said nothing to Maurine, who went about blissfully setting up our house—a happy newlywed. The dean called me back in and told me, "Well, you've got an IQ high enough to keep you here, so that's not it. We made a call to another school we have a relationship with in North Carolina. They have a fine medical program and they agreed to take you there to complete your education. You'll have to put in some extra work to catch up, but they said they'll work with you."

North Carolina? I was setting up my first marital home a few blocks away in Brookline, Massachusetts. Now I had to pick up and move to another state? My head spun. I should have been thankful. *I'd failed!* This guy was doing me the biggest favor in the world, and yet it still seemed like a crushing defeat. I'd have to tell Maurine and my parents and they'd all think I was a failure.

"Or …?"

The dean looked perplexed. What an ingrate I was! "Or … you can stay here and repeat your first year."

"I'll stay here."

"You may want to go home and think about it."

"No, I'll stay here."

"You'll have to keep seeing a psychiatrist. We still think you have some problems."

"I'll see a psychiatrist." The whole psychiatrist thing was making me laugh. A shrink? A shrink was going to tell me what? That people have to study to get through medical school? I knew what I was doing wrong. I suffered from no mental illness. But as best as I could make out, this was Harvard's hangup, not mine. They simply could not understand how one of their own could be such an abysmal failure. I had to have had a breakdown of some sort. That was the only answer they would accept as a reflection on their own institution. What a crock! The problem was me, not them, and not because I was mentally ill, but because I was immature and ridiculous.

I began the sessions immediately and gave them what they wanted. I did not tell them I partied too much and drank too much. They'd ask about my upbringing and I'd allow them to believe I had a tough father who never loved me—garbage like that. I wasn't serious at all about the process. I would have copped to anything so long as they allowed me to stay in school. But I never told them the truth. They didn't seem to want to know the truth. And if they didn't want to face the truth, then neither did I.

Facing Maurine was the thing I dreaded most, but I figured I could not put on a charade that I had moved on with my second year of medical school when I was, in fact, repeating my first. Not that the thought hadn't crossed my mind, but the more I thought about it, the more I realized there was no way I could pull it off. She and everyone else in my family knew how long it took to get through medical school and eventually they would have realized I was there one year too many. They weren't stupid.

Maybe it was because we were newlyweds and she loved me so, but overall she was pretty nice about the whole thing. It rocked her, no doubt about that, but she gathered herself and said, "Well, at least you're still in school and you're still here. It could be worse. I don't feel like moving and I'd hate if you had to give up medicine completely, so all in all this isn't so bad." She asked me some questions—all the basic ones—but she didn't blow a gasket. She told me she was hurt I didn't tell her right away, but it was a small, melancholy reaction rather than an explosion. I told her I was confused, that I didn't know exactly what to tell her since the whole thing was so up in the air. But that was a poor excuse.

I did not drown my sorrows prior to telling Maurine about my dilemma. No doubt I was in a state of depression, but I did not try to anesthetize myself. Perhaps I was afraid of losing control and blurting out the truth to her. After I told her, I felt like a weight had been lifted off of me. I should have still been depressed but I wasn't; I was relieved. But that did not seem to be cause for drunken response either. I actually drank very little that summer. Outside of my educational situation, I was a new husband living with the girl of my dreams. Maurine intoxicated me. She got me higher than a kite.

We got in the car together to make the trek back to Brockton to tell my parents. We were both yawning, which is not as strange as it sounds, as people often yawn when they are nervous and tense.

My father was not as mellow about it all as Maurine had been. He ranted, raved, and screamed. "Do you realize how much medical school costs? And now you want me to pay for an additional year?" The walls shook and I sat there and took it. What else could I do? Which is exactly what I told him.

"What do you want me to do *now*? I'm going back and I'm going to fix it. They're giving me a second chance and I'm taking it. I'll work harder. Case closed."

Once he blew it all out of his system, we moved on. My mother stayed reticent throughout the whole thing—she would never fight with my father in front of me—and went along with what we decided. No one, including me, even discussed me going to North Carolina. For me, it was mostly arrogance. I was a Harvard man. Going to North Carolina—or anywhere else, for that matter—was akin to being demoted, and I was not taught to accept demotion, not after Harvard. Harvard now, Harvard forever. For Maurine and my family, it was more an issue of staying close to home. I was a local boy from a close-knit family. The greater Boston area was my home. This was where I belonged. We would all rather I repeat a year at Harvard than move away.

I believe it turned out to be a wise decision beyond ego, though. I didn't deserve to pass, and going to North Carolina would have been passing. Were I to have done that I might have failed there, too, because I simply did not digest and comprehend the material I should have learned in my first year. Who was I fooling?

For the rest of his life, my father made sure I knew that I had embarrassed him. He may not have screamed about it anymore, but it lingered over our relationship. If we didn't like one another before, we certainly didn't like each other now. I went out of my way to avoid him despite how geographically close we were.

He bought a home in Marshfield, Massachusetts, overlooking the ocean. He asked that I help him put on an addition that summer. When I arrived, he handed me a shovel and had me start digging a foundation. New Hampshire may be the granite state, but that ground in Marshfield felt like granite. My dad stood over me and watched me struggle. I'd look at him and he'd look at me. I knew this was no accident. He wanted to watch me dig ditches. That's what he thought of me now. I was nothing more than a ditch digger. By the time I drove back home to Boston my hands were bloodied and blistered. Maurine was aghast. "How are you supposed to do lab work? Your hands are going to take weeks to heal. Why do you let him do this to you?"

I knew the answer. I was being punished. I'd been raised to fear him and respect him, but not to love him. If he called, I came. If he asked for something, it was my obligation to give it to him. But now, now that I was no longer the golden boy, it was more abusive. I knew I would never again please him, no matter what I did. I had failed.

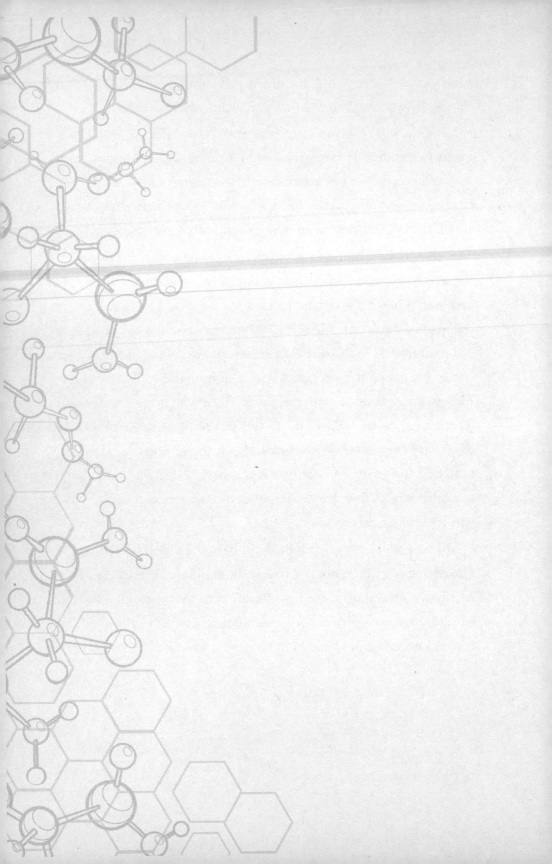

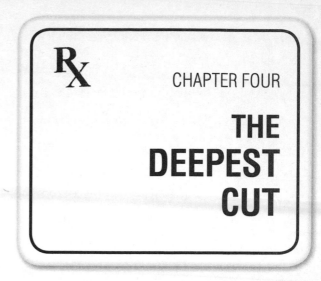

CHAPTER FOUR

THE DEEPEST CUT

Repeating a class is embarrassing enough. Repeating an entire school year is mortifying. Luckily, college and medical school are more spread out socially than grade school and high school. Different people took different classes in different sections at different times of day, and since I didn't have a ton of friends at medical school anyway, not a lot of people noticed I was a repeater; they just presumed I didn't have class with them that year. Doing first year all over again was pretty easy. I may have failed it once

but I was always intellectually capable; I just didn't care enough
my first time through. Now I had the fear of God in me, as well
as the enthrallment of a new marriage and the expectations of my
beautiful new wife. I wasn't going to blow it again.

Maurine worked as a teacher that '68 to '69 school year, but lo
and behold, she got pregnant and was unable to begin the 1969
school year—my official second year of medical school (although
it was the third year I'd physically been there). Was the pregnancy
planned? Yes and no. We wanted children early—it was the thing to
do at the time—although we also knew it would be tough with me
being in school and her being unable to work for a while. Still, we
were happy—two kids too much in love to notice how impractical
we were being. My answer to everything was, "When I become a
doctor, everything will be fine." Even with my early failure I never
once doubted I'd become a doctor, and with being a doctor came
all the benefits America could provide.

By getting Maurine pregnant, I handed my father even more
power to make me miserable. He was paying my tuition and he was
also handing me $300 a month, which covered our $180 a month
rent and a little more to live on. He also came by with groceries on
occasion, which was certainly appreciated—until we tried eating
them. For a man who grew up in a grocery store and knew good
food from bad, the man brought us things I knew he himself would
never eat if he were on a deserted island, like premade hamburger
patties that likely contained more cardboard, sawdust, and pink slime
than meat. I always chalked it up to passive-aggressive behavior on
his part.

If repeating my first year didn't wake me up and make me grow
up fast enough, looking into the eyes of my baby daughter Katie in

November of 1969 certainly did the trick. Like the first time I saw Maurine, I was transfixed. I literally swooned. No greater love hath man than this. Her big blueberry eyes hypnotized me. I really didn't think I would like kids so much. Wearing my white coat, I was able to breeze past the maternity-ward nurses and visit her as often as I wanted, and I *always* wanted to see her. Back then, babies and mothers got a much longer hospital stay, and medical students like me didn't have to flash our IDs a hundred times to prove we weren't child abductors.

Eighteen months later I was back in the nursery again, Maurine having borne me twins, Nicole and Amanda. Here I was, still in medical school, and I had three daughters and a wife with no ability to care for them and hold a full-time job at the same time. We defined young and crazy, and yet we were never so happy. Nicole and Amanda were every bit as beautiful and perfect as Katie, and I'm not just saying that because they're mine. They came out so healthy and well-developed for twins, who are frequently underweight and more prone to developmental issues that require a longer hospital stay. When it came to kids, I'd struck it lucky three times in a row, so much so I probably took it for granted.

The twins were born the day internships were announced at the end of medical school. I wanted to stay in Boston to work at the Peter Bent Brigham (now Brigham and Women's) Hospital. The Brigham, like Mass General, had a relationship with Harvard Medical, and both had some of the finest doctors in the world.

By this time I'd done my rotations and seemed to have finally found my niche in life in surgery. Up until then, I'd gone into medicine for almost all of the wrong reasons, the only shining light being my empathy for my mother and her chronically poor health.

I was in it for the prestige and the money, pretty much the reason kids nowadays go to Wall Street. But surgery—it was like falling in love with Maurine and my girls. Something just clicked, as if I'd suddenly found myself in the place where I was always meant to be. I may not have had the world's most mechanical mind, but surgery isn't always like that. It's not pure physics or three-dimensional engineering. It's so much more, and it spoke to all of my best skills and interests. I loved the idea of seeing a problem and solving it creatively. Finally, I'd found a passion, and the Brigham had some of the leading surgical minds in the world, doctors who were not only changing medicine, but also changing attitudes about the field itself. It was an exciting time and it intoxicated me in the healthiest way possible.

This was probably the soberest period of my life, in all the best ways. I went to school and then came home to my wife and family. I loved what I was doing, loved my family, and was scared to death I might screw up again as I did in my first year. Did I miss the party life? Not at all. I would not have come to school with a hangover if my life depended on it. Drinking was never that important. It was a social lubricant, and my social life now was either nonexistent or centered around Maurine and the babies. And I was good with that. I'd never been happier, nor would I ever be so happy again.

In my third and fourth years of medical school I hung out at the Brigham and spoke with the surgeons whenever they would give me the time of day. I wanted to get to know them and I wanted them to get to know me. I stayed after and put in so many extra hours purely out of love for the field. I canceled vacations so I could pick up extra hours. The place started to feel more and more like my home away from home. Paradoxically, for the first time in my life, wanderlust set in. I'd spent my entire life in the greater Boston area. Meeting medical students from all over the world and talking to doctors at places like the Brigham, Mass General, and Beth Israel—another fine Boston-area hospital—who had originally studied hither and yon, I came to discover Boston was not the only game around. Over Christmas break of my final year, I visited San Diego. The hospital at the University of California San Diego (UCSD) was doing some great work in surgery and I wanted to check it out. Up until my visit, all I was looking for was a backup to the Brigham. But once I stood on my hotel balcony and saw people swimming around and tanning outside in late December, I thought, "What, am I crazy?" Who needed another Boston winter? I changed my application and made UCSD my first choice.

Getting your first choice for residency is by no means automatic, but my luck held, and when matches were announced, I got San Diego. I was so excited. Maurine was not. It's one thing to feel tethered to one's family and region for purely emotional reasons, but with three baby daughters in tow, the thought of moving to the other side of the country made her miserable and I should have been more understanding. But I was a chauvinist in a more chauvinistic time. I was going to be a world-famous surgeon and if that meant going to the South Pole or Atlantis under the sea, then that's where we'd all go, dammit.

I packed up the family and drained our bank account, which had been accruing interest on our wedding money and had grown to around $4,000. An internship paid around $8,900 a year, which even then was modest for a family of five, but by then I felt I was well on the road to riches. Surgeons made the big bucks.

I went out early to look around and get us settled. I asked around for the best place to live and everyone said, "La Jolla." Nice enough to say—and true as well—but a hell of an expensive place for a family living on what I was going to be making. But this became the start of another of my future downfalls—the desire for artifice over substance, better known as living above one's means. Spending money was fun—too much fun. I'd spend it when I was bored. Spending money became a stimulant, a drug of its own sort. But they don't tell you about that when people discuss addictive behavior. It doesn't necessarily involve drinking, smoking, or snorting anything. You do, though, use money to buy all those things, but you can also get addicted to using money (or credit) to buy any darn thing that makes your pupils dilate and your heart quiver a little. Spending breaks up life's mundanities the same as any consciousness-altering substance or experience.

Luckily, I found a steal—a rental house with an ocean view for only $400 a month. I went to a department store, got my first credit card, purchased three cribs, and then decorated the rest of the house. I then went to Household Finance and borrowed some more money in order to live an even higher life. The furniture was new, albeit from a discount store, but the address was prestigious and I felt it showed me off as being more than I really was at the time, which I found important. Harvard, perhaps, had given me an ego, and failing my first year of med school had put an "I'll show them" chip on my shoulder, much to my future detriment.

In San Diego I kept up my hard work and sobriety while continuing to be enthralled with surgery. I made a friend by the name of Dale, a brilliant fellow from the University of Chicago, who lived the single life to the hilt, which I envied at times. With

Dale, I fell off the wagon once in a major way. I did not get along very well with my mother-in-law, much as I did not get along with my father. Maurine's mom was coming out to San Diego for Thanksgiving and I didn't think I could bear it. So I invited Dale over and provided him a bottle of Chivas Regal as an inducement, as if a home-cooked Thanksgiving dinner wasn't enough. But I couldn't let the poor man drink alone, so I bought myself a bottle of Wild Turkey. Together we watched football on TV and matched each other shot for shot like a couple of frat boys. Soon, both bottles were empty and Dale and I were passed out on the couch, much to my mother-in-law's disgust and my wife's chagrin. By dinnertime we both stirred enough to join the gathering at the harvest table, only to have poor Dale pass out once more and fall face first into a plate of mashed potatoes. None of my women were amused, although some of the babies may have giggled.

The Thanksgiving incident was an anomaly, though, yet looking back I rue my motivation in trying to dull my unhappiness with alcohol. Life for me was so good; why did I feel the need to blot out even the most minor of discomforts in such a manner? And yet I did.

Professionally, I started specializing somewhat, finding my greatest interest in general surgery, which sounds like a contradiction of terms, yet it is not. General surgery is the gut, the abdomen. I was doing a lot of gall bladder surgeries at Balboa Naval Hospital, and the more I did, the more possibilities I discovered. I had some pretty decent skills.

I began studying under Dr. Orwell, who specialized, ironically, in maladies usually associated with alcoholism. With him I would do portacaval shunts, a procedure fairly common at the time for relieving the increased venal pressure from hardening liver tissue. Dr. Orwell took a liking not only to me, but also to my friend, Dale. On clinic days, Dale and I were sent out to San Diego's version of Skid Row in order to find and deliver our patients. Our studies proved very valuable to the medical community because alcoholic patients were notoriously irresponsible when it came to attending their follow-up visits, so much so that many doctors just let it go. But Orwell wanted to learn more, and so each and every week, out went Dale and I to gather up our drunks so they could be monitored.

Logic would dictate that exposure to such a seamy underbelly of humanity, made so by drinking, would have sobered me up completely, but I compartmentalized it. That was them and I was me. They were sick bastards who couldn't hold a job, lived in the street, and if they had a dime in their pocket, it went straight to the liquor merchant. Me, I was a doctor. None of the above could possible pertain to me, ever. And even when I did stupid things like down an entire bottle of Wild Turkey, I still could not identify. I didn't feel the need to abuse my body that way every day. That, to me, was the difference. So long as I could go a day, a week, or a month without drinking to that level of excess, I proved to myself and the world I did not have a problem. But I was looking at the entire issue through the lens of frequency. I never considered my *motivations* for drinking. That Thanksgiving Day episode would set off bells and whistles at most every rehab center or twelve-step meeting. But I wasn't going to those sorts of places, nor was I speaking with anyone in the addiction or mental health field. I was only dealing with the mechanics of the aftermath of addiction: liver disease and such. And yet while another person might see what I saw and swear off ever drinking a drop again, it never had that effect on me. Pick up a drunken bum in the morning; go out for cocktails that night. No connection at all.

On a beautiful, sunny San Diego Sunday, I had just finished another well-cooked meal courtesy of Maurine. I had drunk nary a drop of alcohol. We had a babysitter over to help with the kids, and she and Maurine had the three of them out for a stroll.

I decided to help Maurine by cleaning up after the meal. I picked up a crystal bowl by the edge. It was a little bottom-heavy. I brought it up to the light because I noticed some water spots on it and I was going to see how I could attend to it. Suddenly, the thing exploded in my hand as if it had been strafed with a bullet. The bottom-heavy piece came down and sliced my right arm. I remember looking up high, not feeling much of anything, and wondering, "What's that red stuff up on the ceiling?" It was blood. I looked down at my arm. It was my ulnar artery, the major artery on my pinky finger side, and it was pumping fast and furiously, squirting fresh blood all over the place like a geyser. I grabbed a towel and put it around my wrist, then somehow staggered out to my car and started it up. I was in a complete daze, from both shock and loss of blood. I began driving, my left hand holding the towel around the bleeder on my right as I attempted to steer with the bleeding hand, since I am right-hand dominant. I was crazed and dazed, driving around the block over and over again, which gives you a window into how discombobulated I was. Finally, I brought the car to a halt on the opposite side of the street from where Maurine was standing with the kids. I didn't want the babies to get upset so I didn't go near them. As Maurine approached she saw I was covered in blood. "I think you're going to have to take me to the hospital."

The babysitter gathered up the children and went into the house to clean up. Amazingly, she thought to gather together all the crystal pieces and preserve them, like some CSI.

I had sliced five tendons in my right hand, cut my ulnar artery, and my ulnar nerve. I was in surgery for nine hours and woke up the next day with my hand and arm in a cast up over my elbow. I would be in that cast for months.

I may have been sober when the accident occurred, but now all I wanted was to drink or take a pill to make all the pain and sorrow go away—not just the physical pain, but the emotional as well. Months later, we would take the shards of crystal to a lawyer, who brought in an expert to examine it, and would bring suit against the manufacturer, a suit that we eventually won to the tune of $180,000. The bowl never should have shattered, but it was improperly annealed, much to my eternal detriment.

Back then, $180,000 should have made me happy. It should have made anyone happy. But 180 million would not have brought any pleasure to my life. After a couple months off I went back to doing research in the lab, which wasn't as taxing on my arm. I went to physical therapy. I had very little feeling in my right hand. What is a surgeon without his hands? I was like a one-armed pianist or guitar player. Worse, since I really couldn't compensate with my opposite hand.

They gave me a ton of painkillers for the injury and I gobbled them up like candy. I honestly was in a lot of pain. I didn't do anything crazy like steal drugs. Since I was dealing with doctors who were friends, I was given a lot more than the usual leeway when it came to asking for more and more frequent scripts. They figured that, unlike "civilian" patients, I knew what I was doing. Also, most doctors prescribe a bit more than the patient really needs, but I always made "all gone" like a good little eater. But the painkillers weren't the crux of what became a problem for me. I was mixing them with liquor and lots of it. And when I didn't have any drugs around, I just drank. And drank. And drank. I was not drinking to be sociable. I wasn't "partying." I was drinking and taking extra painkillers because I was miserable and wanted to die now that I knew I had lost the ability to perform surgery. Not that I thought I could or would drink myself to death, but I did it out of depression, and if a truck had tried to run me over during that period I would have said, "Go ahead; make my day."

After a long layoff, I was encouraged to try my luck in the operating room once more. I stopped drinking and drugging. It was like football all over again. It was time to get back in shape. Yet I never stopped to consider that attitude, but merely accepted it as a healthy one. With a mission in life, I could stay clean and sober. Without a mission, my default mechanism was to become chemically altered, and I was good with that.

Stepping into the operating theater suddenly gave me the shivers. Where once I felt exhilaration and the warm spotlight of stardom, I now felt nothing but dread. I couldn't feel my damn hand, my damn right hand. I no longer had the confidence to do the simplest of procedures. How the hell was I going to shine at this? How could I make this my life's work now? My confidence was shot.

My supervising surgeon was a good man who knew what I'd gone through, knew that I'd been out of the OR for almost a year. He wasn't going to bust my chops, but he couldn't do all the work for me, either. What would be the point? I was there to learn how to be a surgeon, not watch and pretend.

A lot of surgery is done by feel. You go into certain areas blindly. I kept leaning over, trying to see what no one could possibly see. I couldn't feel. Without the sense of touch, all I had were my eyes. But it was ridiculous. It's like trying to drive a car while looking down at your feet. You can't do it, and if you try long enough someone is going to die.

"You can't do that," he said, as patiently as possible.

I panicked. "I know, I know," I said, so damn frustrated. He was right, of course. I could neither see nor feel. What else was left; operating by *smell*? The entire room was now my enemy. I hated the very walls that held up the ceiling. I hated the scrubs, the mask, the lights; I hated everything. I just wanted to get out of there. The room was a betrayal that taunted me.

I stepped out. I ruminated on the event the entire evening at home. I could not sleep. The next day I went into the office of the chief of surgery. "I'm really nervous," I said.

"It's okay," he said. "Stay in the lab for a while."

The man was willing to be patient with me, to let me go at my own pace, but it looked bleak to me. Time had already gone by and my sense of sensation and some of my mobility appeared permanently impaired. Practicing in the lab, I saw no improvement. It seemed like an exercise in futility, like a man with no arms trying to pitch a baseball. There weren't enough years in a life for things to miraculously turn around on their own, nor was there any therapy or surgery that could bring things back to the way they were. I wasn't in denial—those around me were.

My friend Dale came to my rescue with the only solution that made any sense. He had lost interest in surgery voluntarily and switched to emergency medicine. "Skip, why beat yourself up? You're making less than $9,000 a year. I'm making close to $10,000 a month! Log in some ER hours. No one wants to do this battlefield medicine. That's why we get combat pay."

I'd been a lost soul in college, dragged into medicine for all the wrong reasons when my heart wasn't really in it. Then things finally clicked and my heart was pure and it sang with dreams of becoming a great surgeon. I would have done it for free. But now I was back to the lowest common denominator once more—money. All I heard when Dale talked was, "$10,000 a month." He could have described anything; it didn't matter anymore. Emergency medicine is a noble and important thing, but in my mind I was just prostituting myself. My self-esteem was shattered.

I announced my decision to the chief of surgery. I told him, honestly, that the operating room now scared me and I had to move on. "You're making a huge mistake. Take more time. Rehab your hand. Don't give up." But I did give up. It seemed like the only logical thing to do. I was restless and unhappy. He thought that given enough time, I could get back to where I was, but I didn't believe it nor was I willing to be that patient. Dale was out-earning me ten to one, and he didn't have a wife and kids. I'd grown to love La Jolla, but La Jolla is an expensive place to live. I had visions of my kids attending the finest private schools. Yes, I wanted the big nice house and the fleet of cars, but I also felt an obligation to give Maurine and the girls a certain lifestyle, one befitting my Harvard education.

I wasn't happy with my decision; I was resolved. I settled. It was like marrying the ugly girl with the million dollar dowry. I'd had a chance to know real, deep, and true satisfaction and joy. With that gone from my life, as I saw it, all that was left was to skate along the surface of superficial pleasure. It wasn't just the change in vocations. Soon, it became my approach to everything.

CHAPTER FIVE

DOCTOR TO THE STARS

As soon as I got the job working in emergency medicine, we bought a house on Mt. Soledad facing north overlooking the ocean and La Jolla itself. I just as quickly leased a Cadillac convertible—a fire-engine red El Dorado with leather interior and fuel injection. That car was so big and eye-catching, people would literally stare at me as I drove down the street and young boys would chase after me. Shortly thereafter, I added a Porsche 911 to my collection.

Everything was going swimmingly—if I ignored the fact I was spending money like I made it on a printing press in the basement.

But more just kept coming in, so I figured there would never be a point where I'd get caught short. What bank or financial institution back then wouldn't give credit to a doctor? It would be un-American!

With my rise in income came my fourth and last child, a son, Sylvester IV, better known as Chip, who was born just a few hours after the Bicentennial in 1976. Of my children's births, Chip's was the first where I went into the OR with Maurine. Ultrasounds were still fairly new and we never had one done; furthermore, we would not have wanted to know the baby's gender anyway. Thus, when the doctor said, "It's the boy kind," the announcement took me by surprise, so much so I almost fainted, embarrassingly enough, which had never happened to me in a medical setting before. Perhaps I assumed all babies were female.

I celebrated in style, bringing magnums of Dom Perignon to the hospital to share with everyone in sight, although I probably drank most of it myself. We turned many of those empty bottles into lamps, which make me think of that blessed day every time I see them. Chip had it all—including two maids at his beck and call throughout his childhood. More than any of my other children, Chip was truly born with a silver spoon in his mouth, courtesy of his daddy the doctor.

Maurine's sexy younger sister Therese moved out to the west coast to join us and begin a life of her own. She soon took up with Elmer, the owner of some of the biggest and most historic rock clubs in Los Angeles. He was at least thirty years her senior, but being with him was heady stuff, running around with all the big names in Hollywood. In no time, Maurine and I were swept into the scene, without complaint. I may have been a conservative, but I loved rock-and-roll, as did Maurine. Elmer knew the way to a girl's heart included befriending her family, and with his connections to our rock-and-roll idols, he had Maurine and me eating out of his hand. He learned my favorite band was coming to LA to do a special benefit concert and he got us fabulous seats we could have never gotten on our own. That concert was the first time I ever tried cocaine. It knocked my head back but somehow I managed to have one of my few lucid and reflective moments. *This stuff is so good, I know if I do it again, I'll want to do it more and more and more and more and pretty soon I won't be able to stop until my heart thumps out of my chest.* I spent the rest of the night trying mightily, and surprisingly successfully, to avoid doing any more. But it was everywhere.

I had a new, true love in my life—the rock-and-roll party scene. With my new connection, I could go to a concert every night, and I often did. I couldn't get enough. I was addicted.

At the time, I was working in a hospital in the San Gabriel Valley, about 100 miles from La Jolla. I was torn. I didn't want to commute such a long way, but I loved La Jolla and Maurine had put down roots there. Meanwhile, the LA nightlife drew me in and the thought of being far away from it bothered me. A new, nontraditional addiction had its hooks in me. I could have gotten a job at a hospital closer to where I lived, but that would have taken me farther from LA and the music.

Then Elmer made it worse. "I've got a problem, Skip. My headliner for three shows doesn't think he can perform. Sore throat. I've taken him to two of the best ear, nose, and throat guys in LA and they've both told him there's nothing wrong with him. All that did was piss him off. I don't know if it's in his head or what, but

I have three sellouts I'm going to have to make refunds for and I
don't like that a bit."

"So where do I come in?" I said into the phone.

"You're in emergency medicine and this is an emergency. I'll
bring you in to see him. I'm running out of doctors and he claims
his throat is killing him."

I replied, "But, but . . ." yet it was like I was the undertaker
who asked for a favor from the Godfather. He knew not when the
Don would be in to get his payback, but he knew it would happen
someday, and with all the perks I'd been getting from Elmer, I
knew he'd eventually want something in return. In a sense, I was
relieved it wasn't a request for illegal drugs—pharmaceutical cocaine
or something of that nature. But I had no idea what I could do
for a rock star's sore throat that the best ENT guys in Hollywood
couldn't fix.

They buzzed me inside, and my nerves were setting me on edge.
There he was with a cigarette in one hand, a joint in the other, a
whiskey in front of him, and a babe on his lap. I tamped down the
temptation to point out the obvious—a man claiming to have a sore
throat should lay off the smoke and the drink (the babe would be
okay in my book).

I slowly approached him, and he offered me his complaint. I
looked at his throat and saw nothing of consequence. Normally
that would have been the end of it, but I was there at the behest
of a frantic concert promoter, not a hypochondriac patient, so
the dynamic was altered. I stroked my chin and let out a pensive,
"Hmmmm . . ." in order to buy time. I then called a local pharmacy
for a steroidal inhaler . . . that would do absolutely nothing. It would
also do no harm, which is right there in the Hippocratic Oath, so

I was still good with the gods of medicine, but the whole idea was psychological. I was using the ol' placebo effect. I was going to go pick it up myself, but Elmer insisted on sending one of his girls, these beautiful bartenders and waitresses who were every bit as drop-dead gorgeous as any runway model. That gave me more time to hang out and feel like I was part of a rocker's entourage.

I was the guest of honor at the shows that night, getting a big table with buckets of champagne I did not have to pay for, surrounded by all the hottest girls. After the first set, a guy came up to me and said, "They need you backstage." This only made me look like more of a big shot. Sauntering back to the dressing room, my clearly worried patient said, "I know you said to only take so much of this stuff and it would last for a long time. But I have another set and I'm worried my throat is getting tender again. Can I do more?" I knew there was no harm, yet I acted like I was twisting in the wind before finally saying, "Okay, but just this once." Filled with confidence, he did a great second show and I had somehow saved the day. He even gave me a shout-out from the stage, which really made me feel like king of the world. I ended up spending the night in Elmer's house, which was a gorgeous mansion that was also used as a set in the movie, *Less Than Zero*, about the opulent decadence of LA nightlife.

I had illusions of, perhaps, becoming the "house physician" for Elmer at his various LA clubs after that, but there were already guys more local than I for that gig. Still, I enjoyed seeing all the shows—any act I ever wanted to see—and even getting backstage from time to time. It got me thinking this could be a type of job in general—rock star medicine—if not with Elmer, then perhaps somehow, somewhere.

I had to bone up on other aspects of my medical training. I had so dedicated myself to surgery I'd let other things slip past me. Now, determined to do my best at emergency medicine, I had to get my skills together in other areas and learn to look at cases from a different perspective. I had to be a medical doctor first and a cutter second, unlike a scalpel-happy surgeon. Odd as it sounds, I can't help but think my infrequent experiences treating rock stars for Elmer provided me with a bit of positive incentive.

I was driving two hours each way to work and working twenty-four-hour shifts sixteen days a month. This was just the work-work, not the fun-work, which I did for Elmer. It was a killer schedule and not one conducive to a happy family life. Add to that my penchant for rock-and-roll nightlife and it was a less-than-pretty picture for a young wife like Maurine, who had her hands full with four little babies. To make it worse, I was an old-fashioned guy in many ways— all the wrong ways. As the man of the house, I expected to be loved, worshipped, and adored. My word was law. And being a doctor, an occupation second only to God, made me even more insufferable. Lastly, there is no question that emergency medicine is about saving lives. Saving lives! What a chip *that* put on my shoulder. God only rested on the seventh day so I could take over!

Marriage, every marriage, is a joining of the best and worst of both parties involved. We all have our own personal quirks—things most would find intolerable in others—and we combine that with someone else's, which makes for one hell of an emotional cocktail. In the end, it doesn't matter who's right and who's wrong more often on average; the situation is still combustible and more than a bit off-kilter. Because of my hours, because of the travel, I needed the rock-and-roll nightlife to blow off steam and relax. *Dumb move*, and not the sort of thing I would advise to someone trying to make a marriage and family work. Because of all this, I spent many a night back up in LA, not even bothering to come home to Maurine and the kids—another antifamily move. Then, when I came home, Maurine would spend most of the time yelling at me for never being home. There's the illogic! It mattered not that she was right; being greeted by this made me think, "Wow, I was just at a great concert and now I'm being chewed out. I think next time I'll just stay at the club." If something feels good, we're drawn to it. If something feels bad, we run away from it. It's the definition of selfishness, irresponsibility, and immaturity, but it is primal, and at the end of the day, we are all primitives deep down inside. It is that aspect of our psyche that makes us do the worst things we do.

Our marriage was beginning to tatter. If my hours weren't bad enough, now I was avoiding coming home more and more because I felt it was an inhospitable place—*because* of my hours. Talk about a circle of discontent.

One day I came home and all my stuff was out in the driveway. This was a wake-up call. Maurine accused me of being unfaithful and even though she had no direct evidence, guys who don't come home at night are prone to incite such suspicions, especially when they've got a few bucks in their pocket and carry matchboxes from all the hottest nightspots around—places where singles mingle.

Instead of begging for forgiveness, young Dr. God simply gathered up his stuff, threw it in his Porsche, and headed back to LA. I got myself an apartment in Westwood, near the UCLA campus, and looked forward to the single life. The kids would come up and see me, and I would come visit them from time to time, but for a year, Maurine and I were separated. I felt I'd tried to explain myself quite well during the time we were still living together, but I failed to ever see her point of view. That was my immaturity. For as much as I loved the kids when they were first born and in diapers, now something else held my attention more—being a big-shot celebrity doctor, hanging around with rock stars.

Around this time, the group I was affiliated with at the hospital where I worked had their contract come up for renewal. We either had to take a significant pay cut or lose out to a competitor. We let the other company take the contract. It made us feel good about ourselves, maintaining our professional pride. Of course, it also left us all unemployed, not that doctors generally have trouble picking up work. But it did mark a milestone in my life, one where I could make major changes, untethered to a particular situation.

This was a massive moment for me. It was a point where Maurine and I could have severed all legal ties and gotten a divorce, or else it could be a sign it was time for me to make some changes and recommit to our marriage. I decided to recommit, and although angry, she was loyal and decided to take me back. A big point in the negotiations was that I had to take a job closer to where we lived. She also preferred we get away from LA, which she now felt symbolized everything that had gone wrong with our relationship. Yes, she loved rock-and-roll as much as I did, but you can find rock-and-roll anywhere. This was about the nightlife, the party life, and while Maurine was no stay-at-home stick-in-the-mud, she wasn't as addicted to the scene as I. She was a mother and had that natural instinct to be with her brood. Me, I was a young guy who'd already gotten somewhat bored with domesticity and longed for the jetsetting life. But now I had to choose one or the other, so I chose Maurine. Or so we both thought.

We decided to head back east, to Massachusetts. If LA and California had come to symbolize for Maurine all that had gone wrong between us, perhaps a return to our roots would bring back the Skip she had fallen in love with. We bought a house on Cape Cod, near the Merchant Marine Academy, in an area called Gray Gables, right on the water. We moved into the house before I even had a job. But again, as a doctor, you don't worry about things like that. You're a hot commodity and money is always just around the corner.

I got a job at a hospital in Attleboro, Massachusetts. Like our situation in California, it was not just around the corner, but the hour drive each way was through Nowheresville, so there were no hot nightclubs to distract me from coming straight home.

But then something developed. Close to the hospital someone decided to build an outdoor amphitheater named Great Woods. Amazingly, rock-and-roll would cross my life's path once more. The head of the hospital called me in, as head of emergency medicine, and asked what I thought of us having some sort of presence at Great Woods, perhaps as their go-to medical facility. I went to the developers and they gladly brought me aboard to help them design and lay out a first-aid center. Meanwhile, I came upon some great emergency room doctors who happened to be looking for placements in the greater Boston area. Ours may not have been the most prestigious hospital in the state, but it was a state that drew a lot of talent and I was able to surround myself with some great doctors in my department, which made me look good.

The idea the hospital and the Great Woods people had was that we would be primarily serving the fans who came to see the outdoor shows. I, on the other hand, still had stars in my

eyes, courtesy of Elmer, with whom I still kept in touch. I got
a few names and made it known we could also service the acts
themselves, if they needed us. It didn't necessarily have to be for
emergency work—heck, a lot of these musicians liked to find a
local chiropractor or what have you when they were on the road. I
wanted to be the man who took care of their needs.

The rock-and-roll acts started to come in. Even with stars in my
eyes, I tried to keep very professional when it came to patient care.
There but for the grace of God goes any doctor who forgets his
main job is to follow his oath rather than be a sycophant to a star.

Some of the musicians were on medications I couldn't just take
their word for, so I had to call their primary care doctors in order
to confirm the diagnosis and care protocols. I also insisted on taking
blood levels and any other pertinent test to make sure I wasn't being
scammed. I figured the fellas would think I was being a pain in the
ass, but instead they seemed to respect me for it. I wasn't busting
chops; I was giving them first-class care.

Along with backstage access, I was also guaranteed a handful of
great free seats to every show. By this time my kids were starting to
follow music and they loved to make the concerts a family outing. I
even brought them backstage from time to time, much to their delight.

Between LA and Great Woods, I'd found a spark I hadn't felt
since surgery. I loved rock-and-roll. I loved the music and the people
who made it. Emergency medicine was just a means to an end. If I
could have been named podiatrist to the stars, I probably would have
signed on for that gig as well. The medicine was no longer the thing.
The type of patients was what got me out of bed each day.

I don't know what this says about my pleasure centers or my
values at that point in my life. Pretty shallow, one might think. But

compared to how I felt during my down periods, such as after my accident, this all felt pretty darn good to me, and so the things I did, healthy and unhealthy, I did out of a sense of joy and having been blessed. Never, though, did I stop for true personal reflection. When good things are going on around you, why ask why? Furthermore, why ask what it all means, and what you're doing with all that joy? My life was becoming more and more like the day Chip was born. These were the champagne days—and like that day, I was the one consuming most of the bubbly.

I was up for the position of chief medical officer at the hospital. The whole thing was rather political, which I didn't object to. Coming from Harvard and surrounded by some pretty well-to-do characters, I'd learned how that game was played. I'd wine and dine the decision-makers and do a lot of backslapping. On the other hand, my big Brockton mouth got me in trouble more than once. I'd grown up opinionated and stubborn and never quite learned to shut up when doing so would have been in my best long-term interests. I was also drinking a lot, which loosened my tongue even more, as well as the thermostats on my temper. I never showed up to work impaired, but it's never a good idea to be the drunken loudmouth at the end of the bar surrounded by coworkers, yet that's what I became.

There's an oddity about drinking. When you do it in a dive bar, surrounded by the dark denizens of depressed dourness, you feel like a loser and you face your demons as such. When you're downing drink after drink at The Harvard Club or some other ritzy joint, surrounded by the high and mighty, you get just as drunk but you feel like a winner. I felt like a winner, but I drank like a loser, and no matter where you drink, when you do too much, you become a loser.

When the vote for chief medical officer was taken, I lost by one vote. One vote. I heard the murmurs that those who voted against me mentioned my drinking and tied it together with my sometimes irascible manner. Me, I felt they were two separate issues, but when something smells like a goat, tastes like a goat, and brays like a goat, it's probably not a fish.

From there, things went downhill fast. A new CEO took over the hospital and she and I locked horns continuously. Now when I drank, I drank mad—which differs from drinking happy or drinking sad, but only in regard to motivation. In each and every case, I consumed the same amount of alcohol, and in each case I felt justified. So long as I could still work, I was good. That was my eternal mantra.

Eventually, I got so angry one day, I threatened to quit. And so they let me. I was still full of myself and felt completely justified in holding to the opinions I had regarding the running of the hospital that led to my divorce from the place. Nonetheless, I was now unemployed. It mattered little to me, excepting the fact that it took from me the thing that gave my life its spark—rock-and-roll. I knew I'd be employed again or else I'd strike out somehow on my own. I was still a doctor, a young doctor, and there were no official black marks upon my reputation. The bastards weren't going to keep me down.

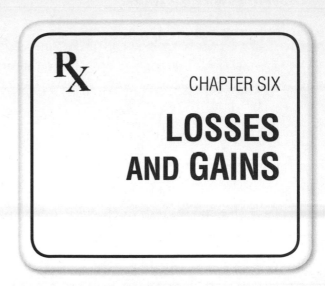

CHAPTER SIX

LOSSES
AND GAINS

I may have butted heads with administrative types, but I had
good relationships with my fellow doctors, as well as the nurses and
assistive staff wherever I worked. You know the big roll of paper
that's used to cover an exam table? A staff member unwound a few
feet of paper from one of the rolls and wrote up a petition asking
my boss to reconsider and do whatever was necessary to keep me,
and nearly every employee in the hospital signed it. It was touching,
but my foot was already out the door and I wasn't coming back
unless my boss resigned instead, which wasn't about to happen.

I picked up hours here and there—when you're a doctor, you're always in demand. Along the way, I started hearing about medical weight-loss clinics, which had become the new rage. Me, I was fifty pounds over my fighting weight, but I wasn't thinking in terms of getting rid of my paunch; I was thinking dollar signs.

I went to a seminar sponsored by the number two company in the business at the time—I won't drop names, but these were meal-replacement milkshakes, which grew to be quite a fad. I liked the taste of their product more than that of the number one company. Either way, it was new and I was getting in on the ground floor, so to speak. The idea was to get people to fast for as long as was appropriate for their weight by replacing their meals with protein shakes. While they were losing weight, we taught them better nutrition so when they got back onto real food, they would make healthier choices. All in all, the program worked, as long as you worked the program. If it ever failed, it was for the same reason most programs fail—noncompliance. It would be years before I would apply this common sense to my own life. Food can be very much like a drug. The problem is, unlike many other addictive substances or behaviors, food does have a positive value; you do have to eat. Also, exercise must be a lifetime commitment.

I didn't want to learn about this program so I could administer it at some other hospital, watching the hospital make all the profits while I was nothing more than an employee. I'd been around a bit by now and saw the doctors who were living large were the ones who thought entrepreneurially. But to open a business you needed to put up some money—money I didn't have, since I spent it all as soon as I got it.

Anyone who says most colleges are created equal never went to Harvard. It's not just the education, it's the connections. By now, guys I'd lived with, studied with, and played ball with were conquering the world. One was an old teammate of mine by the name of Patrick. I'm not privy to his personal finances, but between his investments in restaurants, hotels, advertising, ski resorts, horse tracks, and movie theaters, he's probably worth around a billion dollars.

Patrick gave me the seed money to open a private weight-loss clinic. Why should the hospitals make all the money? I took it private, with visions of dollar signs floating over my head. Patrick was already involved in so many other businesses that the investment I needed was merely lint from the lining of his pockets. He didn't even feel the need to oversee the operation—too small. Besides, I was good ol' Skip, his teammate and a fellow Harvard man. Of course I could take that investment and make it soar. It's what we Harvard guys do.

With Patrick backing me, I then opened a second clinic in Cambridge, then quickly opened a third, backed by Lou, another Harvard teammate, in a big, beautiful skyscraper he built in Boston. In six months, I went from nothing to having three offices spread across eastern Massachusetts. I was on a roll.

We would put out advertisements inviting people to a dog-and-pony show at our clinics and we'd be flooded with attendees. Some were beautiful women who felt they were only ten or fifteen pounds away from looking "just right," despite looking great as they were. It mattered not. If you came through our door, most likely we would put you on the fast, so long as it was not dangerous medically. It wasn't medicine; it was commerce, and so long as we didn't harm anyone—and we didn't—we were good to go. And with it being administered by a doctor in a medical environment, it carried the seal of medical approval. Everybody bought in.

It grew too large too fast. My ambition got ahead of my ability to manage. I was in over my head even from the medical and scientific side. Nutrition wasn't my bag, nor did it hold much interest for me. I contacted a guy who was a professor at Harvard and the chief nutritionist in the Harvard medical system. He had four or five clinics of his own that were far better run than mine. I proposed forming a partnership with him, but we just couldn't come to an agreement.

Meanwhile, I was drinking heavily. What the hell was I doing in the weight loss business? I felt stupid, so I tried to drink away the pain. Even after learning all about this weight loss stuff and opening all these offices, I was now around seventy-five pounds overweight myself. I hadn't lost an ounce. Of course, I also wasn't working the system, but that was beside the point. It became a perfect symbol for this chapter of my life. I was a fraud. I'd get up in front of audiences and give my spiel about how the program worked. When someone would ask why I wasn't built like a Greek god, I'd laugh and say, "You should have seen me before I started this program!" *It was a lie*! But hey, think about the people you see on TV who've just lost 150 pounds. Most of them are still huge. I played the same game. Only if they knew me well could they know I was full of crap. But the lying wore me down, and so I drank. The fact I was playing the huckster wore on me as well. Is this what I went to Harvard for? To lie to suckers like a common thief, like a sideshow carnie?

Maurine helped me with a few big leads. She found herself at the same beauty parlor with the wife of a very successful entrepreneur named Saul. He was the CEO of an athletic apparel company. Saul's not a heavy guy, but like anyone who's in the public eye and has money to spend, he carries a healthy load of vanity and the thought of losing fifteen or twenty pounds appealed to him, so Maurine gave his wife my card. That very night, he called me and asked if I could come see him. When you're the CEO of a global corporation, you don't go to clinics; clinicians come to you. But he told me he'd make it worth my while. "I have a bunch of friends in the same boat. I'll have them all in my boardroom at 7:00 a.m. If we like what we hear, you can sign us all up."

I grabbed my pretty nutritionist, as well our male nurse and a ton of shake samples. When I walked in, I faced about a dozen of the most powerful people in Boston, none of them morbidly obese, but all in search of the newest medical treatment to lose a few pounds. As I was just starting my sales pitch, one guy interrupted and asked, "What are your credentials?" I said, "I went to Harvard College and Harvard Medical School." Before I could finish the thought, Saul said, "That's all we need to know." Part of the deal, and the one part that salved my physician's soul—what little I still clung to—was I insisted anyone who started the program have blood drawn, get a physical, and get hooked up to an EKG so I could determine whether they were healthy enough to go on a fast. Saul was the typical take-charge, no nonsense captain of industry. "I don't know about the rest of you, but I'm ready to start right now." Everyone else, of course, followed suit. When a billionaire says something is the smart thing to do, few people argue.

Saul invited me to accompany him into his private office to complete his physical right then and there. As you can imagine, his office was splendid, but that's not the part I remember the most. I helped him off with his jacket. I'm a doctor. I'm not a poor man. But I had never before nor have I since held a garment in my hand that was so luxurious. From a distance, it looked like any other well-tailored, well-made suit jacket. But touching it—when do we ever touch other people's clothing?—blew my mind. It just felt so . . . expensive. Like more-than-the-cost-of-my-car expensive. Decades later, I will never forget how that suit felt in my hand. It paralyzed me. It represented something I wanted, yet I felt I would never achieve.

I did similar meetings with people—all big shots. This enterprise went on for about a year or two, but I just couldn't make it work financially. When you loathe what you do, how well can you do it? I wasn't practicing medicine; I don't know what the hell I was doing. Was I a businessman? Entrepreneur? Liar? Clown? Finally, I saw no way of saving the operation from bankruptcy except to sell to a competitor, who at least had a passion for the business. Selling gave me enough money to help repay most of Patrick's investment so I could at least look him in the eye once more. But here were Patrick and Lou, super-successful guys I'd played ball with, and here I was, borrowing money and asking favors of them, ostensibly to help make them more money, as if I were their equal as a man and a provider, and I was neither. If America measures a man's worth in dollars, I was so far behind these fellows they couldn't even find me in their rearview mirrors. Patrick's dad was a cop. His background was no different than mine—we came from working class guys. And yet he was way up there and I was far below him. That killed me. It put me inside a bottle.

Patrick and Lou were graduates of Harvard Business School. Back when I was at Harvard College, we used to joke that the really smart guys went to Harvard Medical, the above-average guys went to Harvard Law, and the slackers who couldn't cut it intellectually went to the business school. Yeah, right. These guys made me feel like that entire perception was upside down.

I had lost my compass. After losing the ability to perform surgery, I simply could not find myself. I would have been a surgeon for free; I swear. I loved it so. I was saving lives. After that, even doing emergency room medicine never quite gave me the same sense of satisfaction. Satisfaction comes from within, and one man's trash is another man's treasure. Some guys lived and breathed emergency room work. I didn't. It still saved lives, but it didn't rev my engines. I did it for the money. Now I was selling milkshakes— for the money. What next? How much lower could I go? My only thoughts were on the dollar signs, which is where my priorities got completely screwed up.

I looked at guys like Saul and Patrick and Lou, and I wanted to cry. I could never succeed in their world, the business world, like them. My mind didn't work like theirs did. Saul crystallized it for me one day. He said, "You doctors are never going to make serious money at this." At the time, I thought I was doing well. I'd opened my three clinics and thought things were going up, up, and away. But months before it would dawn on me I wasn't going to make a go of it, Saul already had the whole situation analyzed. "You need to do volume. This business model of yours, it's small-potatoes." I had no idea what he was talking about. A few years later, what he meant was on every grocery shelf in America: Slim-Fast.

If he'd wanted to do it himself, Saul could have pulled it together, but he was busy with his other enterprises. Me, if I'd had the acumen he had, I would have asked him more questions and done it myself. But I didn't. Instead, I argued with him. "You need a doctor involved. It's by prescription."

"You can get around that. What you need is for this stuff to literally be in vending machines, everywhere you turn."

That didn't sit well with me, so I forgot about it. But some other guy took what we doctors were doing and decided the way to make serious money was to mass produce the meal replacement shakes, make it available without a prescription, and have it so every person in the country could go to the corner store and buy it. What I'd been doing was only affordable to the fiscal elite. That's too small a market. Saul knew this, knew it instinctively. I didn't, or I could have been the Slim-Fast guy. Instead, I was just a doctor who had to sell his three offices in order to keep his head above water.

I hated to lose debates like that. I wasn't used to it. I was supposed to be the smartest guy in the room, in any room I occupied. But there are all sorts of intellect and this was where I had no natural talent. I'd grown up assuming it was all about test scores—math problems and word definitions. Little blue ribbons for finishing first. The guys who made billions weren't necessarily the best in math, chemistry, or English. What they knew was a different way of looking at problems, and it drove me nuts because I didn't have it and didn't know where to get it.

Right before I sold my clinics I called Sid and Jenny Craig, who would become billionaires in the diet business. We kept up a correspondence for a while, but I let it go instead of following through and working with them. I was like the guy being offered stock options in Apple or Microsoft or IBM at their inception and saying, "No thanks." Those Harvard Business School guys never would have made that mistake. Hanging around with them was like hanging out with the rock stars, but it affected me differently. I never really aspired to be Keith Richards. I never claimed to have an ounce of musical talent, so being with rock stars never made me feel low. But as I saw it, going from nothing to billions was about smarts, which I thought I had. Apparently, I didn't, and that killed me a little. When I hung out with those guys, I'd retreat into myself at certain points and think, "I'm not on their level. I'm like an employee to them. Yes, I know more medicine than they do and they realize and respect that, but they respect millions of dollars even more and I'll never have that." The more time I spent with them, the more a little bit of me died inside.

And so I drank. When I drank, I was smart again. I was rich. My future was rosy as could be. And when drinking makes you feel that good about yourself, and your sober hours make you feel so badly, was there any choice to be made?

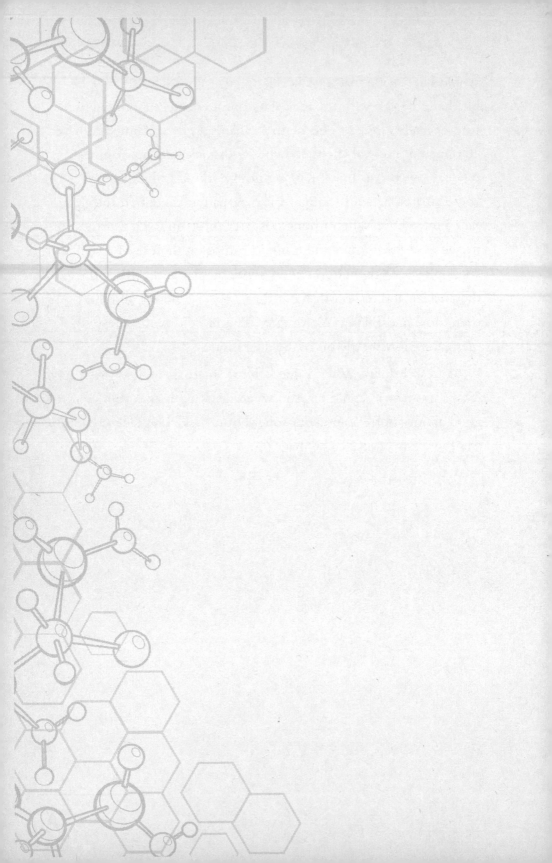

IDLE HANDS, BULGING WITH CASH

Moving back to Massachusetts was a good move for my marriage. I had created havoc in my relationship with Maurine while we lived in California but now, with the change of coasts and the passing of years, things had settled into a comfortable and more acceptable pattern. I was still not the perfect husband but I was, in her eyes, a bit better. Tolerable. But now Massachusetts held nothing for me professionally or emotionally. The end game with the weight-loss clinics had left me emotionally miserable and I was searching everywhere for a solution. Never did I seem to turn inward, but instead felt the answers lay in some external realm.

I had really enjoyed living in California and thought perhaps with my growing maturity (or what I perceived as maturity) a move back there would rekindle my soul. Maurine was skeptical, but outside of the mistakes of my personal choices, she had an affinity to the place as well. I called up a few contacts I still had out there, and, as would be expected, finding a job was not very difficult. But that's all it was—a job. Not a career, not a passion, but a job. It was actually a step down career-wise, but that didn't seem to matter much. I was still in medicine and still pulling in the kind of money doctors are used to. But depression lingered over me whenever I sat still long enough to allow it into my brain. I could not be further from the career track captains of industry were on. They employed people; I was an employee. And when I got depressed, I drank.

I got a position in a clinic around Burbank, near Disney Studios. Here I was, close again to the LA club scene, but this time the whole family and I rented a place near where I worked so there was no excuse for staying out all night and sleeping away from home because of a long commute. Burbank morphed into Glendale, but again, it was all around LA and close to where we lived.

I was no longer in any level of management. I was a grunt taking care of every kind of patient who came through the door. I'd been spoiled for a few years, having had a lot of administrative duties prior to doing the weight loss thing, so my hands-on medicine was a little rusty, but it all came back after a few weeks. Meanwhile, when I allowed myself to think about it, I had trouble pushing the thought out of my head that I'd tumbled down the ladder of life a number of rungs while other guys, Harvard educated or otherwise, were climbing ever-higher.

One day while I was picking up hours here and there to augment my primary salary, I found myself alone in a room full of medication. As a doctor, this is like a lawyer finding himself in a courtroom—business as usual. But I noticed some bottles of Vicodin staring me in the face. Never before had I been tempted to mess around with opioids, but suddenly I thought, "I'm in pain, emotional pain. There's a painkiller. Two plus two equals four." I got my hands on a bottle of thirty tablets and downed it in a day. Instant buzz. I was as happy as when I was drunk, maybe even more so. I did this a few more times. I didn't do it every day—I was afraid of getting caught. I didn't have a legitimate reason for taking it. But I did it now and then, and when I did, I did it to excess, knowing that was the quickest way to feel the maximum effect of the drug. Did I think there was anything wrong with me for doing this? Yes. The pills made me feel happy for a short period of time. But I was miserable.

Time was moving along. The girls were growing up and starting to move out and on their own. I was working around LA when the Rodney King riots occurred, which was morbidly exciting if you worked as an emergency-room physician. Truth be told, working helped me through a lot of my unhappiness. I never took my negative feelings out on patients. As soon as I was at work, every patient reminded me of my mother—the reason I went into medicine in the first place. A patient was a patient, no matter his or her station in life or the complaint. I brought over a thousand people back from the dead, so to speak, during my years as an ER doctor. Most of them may not have walked out of the hospital under their own power—or walked out at all—but a significant number did. As of today, I have never been sued for malpractice. I attribute some of that to luck, but I have always kept the good of the patient I am treating as the foremost obligation of the moment. I wore these accomplishments as a badge of honor. It was only when I took off my white coat that I felt a hole somewhere in my heart.

Money started to roll in, as emergency-room medicine was and still is a rather profitable enterprise. After renting for a while, I found a distressed home sale in the Hollywood Hills—a really fabulous place, where several neighboring houses were occupied by celebrities. I borrowed money from Elmer, with whom I reignited a friendship, in order to close the deal. This was my typical MO—I was rarely patient enough to wait until I could actually buy things on my own. I was always spending not only last week's paycheck, but also this week's and next week's as well. We ended up living in that place for only about six months. Like most deals that sound too good to be true, this one was rife with legal issues and other hidden dilemmas and it was becoming more and more apparent we'd have to spend too much money in order to straighten out the ownership issues to get old liens off our backs. Meanwhile, the more we talked about it, the more Maurine and I waxed nostalgically for San Diego, many miles to the south. Even though I was hanging around with Elmer again, with the passage of time the LA club scene no longer held as much of an interest to me. No one wants to be the "old guy at the club." I made a few calls and soon I procured a position at a hospital down south and we packed up our things and set about relocating back to La Jolla.

It was a lateral career move. I was still a grunt, which gnawed at me, but few fields pay their grunts as well. I bided my time—which for me is never long—and found a hospital nearby that had shaky emergency-room management. I made a few calls, knew how to talk to administrators, and came away with a contract to staff and run their ER, promising to hire top doctors to work alongside me. I was then able to enter into contracts at other medical sites, and pretty soon I was making more money than I'd ever made before in my life.

I was happy. Check that; I was relatively happy. I should have been happy. I was happy when I was working on patients and I was happy when I drank. When I drank, negative thoughts seemed to disappear. No matter how much you've got, there's always something you're missing and that's when depression sets in.

Because of my mid-six-figure yearly income, I spent almost maniacally. Spending made me happy. Drinking made me happy. It was all primal. They say the difference between humans and animals, or grown-ups and children, is the ability to delay gratification. I had not been able to do that since football. As I viewed it, the super-wealthy guys I'd met on the East Coast didn't delay their gratification. That's where I was dead wrong. If you're worth $800 million dollars, you can see a $10 million dollar house and buy it and it's no big deal. I'd have $100,000, see something I liked that cost $200,000, and I'd immediately buy it. Big difference.

We rejoined the La Jolla Beach and Tennis Club, and again I rubbed elbows with the big shots. Again, I felt adrenalized, yet inadequate. Again, I drank to get over it. If I showed up in a nice car, dressed well, and had a tan, I was treated with similar respect to the men I envied. But while we didn't exactly sit around comparing tax returns, I knew where I stood in that crowd and it wasn't at the top. I'd grown up working-class, but I worked the American dream. I hadn't reached the pinnacle though, not if I was using these guys as a guideline, and that was killing me. Ever since leaving surgery, I measured far too much in dollars and cents. My skewed view was that the two-million dollar guy was happier and more important to the world than the million-dollar guy, even if the two-million dollar guy robbed banks or dealt drugs for a living. I didn't understand myself. I forgot I'd have happily been a surgeon for a pittance of what these "masters of the universe" earned. That was now ancient history.

There were so many psychological layers to my drinking it took on a culture of its own. It wasn't just about drinking to be happy and thinking I was more successful than I was. If I drank while sitting at a magnificent, opulent place like the club, the illusion became even more real. The place was a vacation spa and I was Jay Gatsby. I wouldn't have felt that way at some dive bar. If I ever went elsewhere, it was always to a similarly high-brow place. I took Maurine to lunch in San Francisco and Los Angeles. We frequented fine places. I felt good about myself at The Bistro, the Beverly Hills Polo Lounge, Mr. Chow's, and The Ivy. That's how I blew my money. It made me feel good, yet it also made me feel bad, because if I were at a dive bar, I probably would have been the most successful guy in the room. Instead, I kept driving and flying myself to places where I'd feel inadequate, which would make me want to drink more and thus the cycle continued.

Along with drinking, I ate way too much. I was my own version of Bacchus—a god of wine, overspending, and pizza. I never went to work drunk, so to be happy, I ate. A lot. Suddenly, the weight-loss doctor was over 400 pounds. How ironic. But as with the drinking, I was in denial. Unlike some people, I did not gather all my weight in one place, the stomach. I was more like the Michelin Man—big spare tires where my face, neck, arms, stomach, legs, and thighs should be. Because of this, I actually didn't think I looked too bad. Ha! I'd never looked worse in my life.

A standard visit to my internist informed me that my pancreas was crying out for relief. Morbid obesity was messing terribly with my insulin. This was no longer a vanity issue; it was a health issue. That's when it was suggested I go for weight-loss surgery. I needed relief fast, and besides, I was obviously not doing too well when it came to self-control. They had me go through a psychiatric evaluation prior to the procedure and asked about my drinking habits. I lied; they bought it. They warned me I'd either have to give up drinking entirely after the surgery or else limit myself to, perhaps, half a glass of wine a day at most. Yeah, right. I'd do as I'd pleased, which was exactly the attitude that had exploded my silhouette to 405 pounds.

My mantra through everything was the same: if I wasn't impaired while at work, I was not an addict. I could go in hung-over as hell, but so long as I wasn't taking a nip while on the job, I was cool. When I did the Vicodin, I didn't take them at work so again, I was cool. Eating? Eating certainly doesn't impair the ability to work, so long as you can get out of bed and do what you're paid to do. Eating provides some cover for denial. You don't *have* to drink or take opioids, but you *must* eat.

The surgery worked. I lost weight rapidly, but broke all the rules concerning drinking because, well, I still had all those other issues. And right after the surgery, they gave me Vicodin—legally—for the pain, and the downward drift turned into a steep spiral.

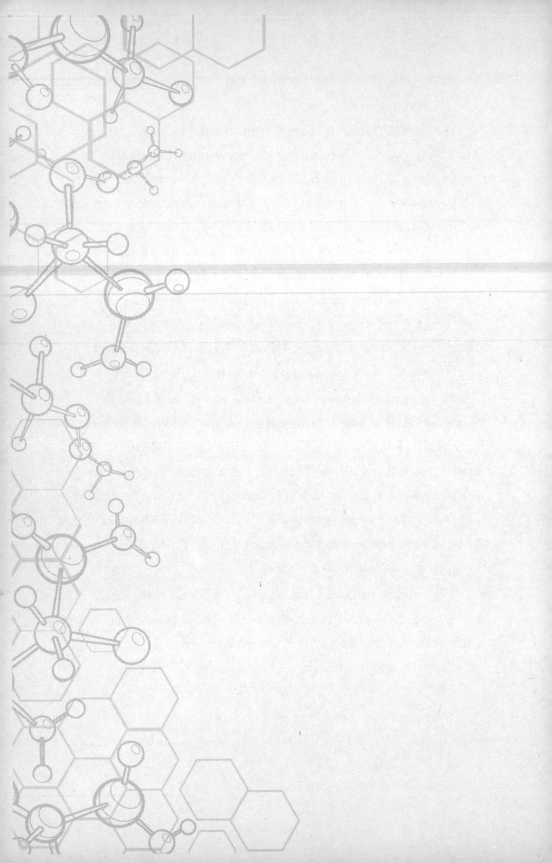

CHAPTER EIGHT

R̲X̲

DOWN IN THE GUTTER, UP ON THE ROOF

Two years. When you first hear a thing like that—that you have a sentence, so to speak, and it has a definite beginning and end—you pull out your calendar, mark down the dates, and start counting off the days. The trouble is, you assume each of those passing days will be normal and pleasant. They aren't. Just ask anyone who ever spent a term in prison. Every single day sucks, and mine did, too.

Denial comes in many forms. When a person loses a job, he or she is apt to say, "I didn't like doing that anyway. Good riddance.

Time to do what I've always wanted, which is (*fill in the blank*)."
At times I tried to look at the loss of my medical license in March
of 1999 as nothing more than that. It left me no choice but to try
something else. The trouble is, it's hard to pursue one's dreams when
one is broke. I had no assets. I had no savings. I'd made a ton of
money—over half a million dollars a year—but I'd spent even more.
With my license gone, the golden goose was killed. Still, I denied it. I
was Dr. Skip and I thought I could succeed at anything I set my mind
to. I could make gold from dirt. Everything was going to be just as it
always had been. There would be no change to my standard of living.
I knew it wasn't true, but I had to believe it, because the honest
voices from deep inside my belly told me I was frightened as hell.

If I had ever angered Maurine before, it was nothing compared
to how she felt about me once I'd thrown away my life for drugs. I
think she would have rather found me dead in bed. A doctor losing
his license over drugs was a man who knowingly flushed away
everything he'd worked for his entire life. It didn't just affect her; it
affected me and everyone who had any relationship to me, past and
present. Her anger wasn't just her feeling sorry for herself; she felt
I had debased myself beyond all recognition, and when you love
someone, you get angry at them for being so self-destructive. I had
punched myself in the nose and neither of us knew for sure if the
bleeding would ever stop.

People around me were shocked at learning of this entire
episode, despite many of them seeing me impaired at one time or
twenty. Just as addicts find themselves in denial, the people around
them often do as well. Dr. Skip couldn't possibly be an addict. He's
a smart guy; he's a good doctor; he's a man to be respected. Even
the main hospital I worked at was in denial. They really liked me.

They liked me so much they tried to go on as if none of this had happened. Sure, I'd lost my license, but I wasn't just a doctor to them. I was doing a lot of administrative things. I ran their ER. Besides, they were having some financial troubles, and they actually owed me money. When people get in debt, they often try to keep the fiduciary relationship going so they have a chance to gradually catch up on their bills, as opposed to breaking off the relationship cold turkey, which usually means having to cough up everything they owe all at once. Owing me money wasn't just for me; it meant I owed money to the doctors who worked under me, so this place owed a lot of people money.

I asked them to keep me employed as an administrative contractor. In my post-narcotics-bender delusions, I figured this was the sort of situation in which I'd land—still involved in medicine, just not seeing patients, which was fine by me. I definitely could have spent two years as a medical administrator. I could have done that standing on my head and smiling.

As I was getting ready to go back to work, the hospital checked with their lawyers. The easiest thing a lawyer can tell you is no. Can we do this? No. Is this legal? No. "No" is easy because it covers their ass. If they're wrong, you didn't do anything anyway, so no one is the wiser. It's only when they tell you something's okay and you do it and it turns out badly that they get in trouble, so "no" is the default mechanism of self-preservation. The hospital lawyers said no, do not hire me back; sever all ties with me, pay me my money as soon as possible, and get out of the Dr. Skip business pronto. This left me immediately adrift. Maurine and I had a little bit of money in the bank, but it in no way measured up to the debts and obligations I'd accrued. I owed lots of money to the IRS, and unlike other creditors, the IRS does little in the way of negotiating and being reasonable.

I tried to clear my head, to put myself in the best possible position to navigate these choppy waters. Our membership at the La Jolla Beach and Tennis Club was paid up until the end of the year so, as crazy as it sounds, I started spending a lot of time there. Unlike the old days, I was not there holding up the bar, pretending to be a big shot. Hell, I was mortified, figuring quite a few people knew about my downfall, which eventually meant they would all come to know. No, I woke up and realized the club was . . . a damn health club! It wasn't just a classy saloon. They had a pool, a fitness center, tennis courts, and a private beach. You could do just about anything there. This was relevant because I felt I needed to get healthy. Getting healthy was more than just detoxing, which I'd already gone through. I needed to exercise, to keep losing weight, to get some air into my lungs and water into and out of my body. I needed to get good healthy endorphins buzzing through my mind and body. And so I went to the club and worked out. It felt good. I didn't talk to many people; a lot of people ignored me or looked down at their feet when they saw me looking their way. It's how people react when someone takes a major tumble in life. They weren't mean enough to come up and call me a jackass, and most of them didn't really know how to properly extend the hand of help and friendship. The easy way out was to pretend I was invisible, which was fine by me because, despite the denial I was in, I was still privately embarrassed as hell. As to my addiction, despite being in my old favorite water hole, I stayed away from the bar at the club and did not partake. I was still physically reeling from the opioid addiction. I certainly knew I could not write any more prescriptions for drugs. Hell, that would have landed me right in jail, which scared me to death. As for drinking, I did as most addicts do, which is I told myself, "Never again," and I held to it awhile, with no real support system or program in place; just me saying it to myself. I took pride in this, and at this stage in my life I needed all the little gold stars on my behavior chart I could muster.

Meanwhile, I tried working things out with the IRS. It became readily apparent the most valuable asset I had was the equity in my house. Selling the house and paying off the remaining debt the house carried would allow me to pretty much pay off the IRS. I did my best to implore the government to, perhaps, leave me with a few dollars upon the sale of the house, my cars, and other valuables I was able to liquidate. But they took it all.

I slowly sank into a massive depression, and despite my return to exercise, I was still a wreck physically. With opioid withdrawal, there is the initial bodily purging, but even after that the body is still not well. Your legs twitch in your sleep and a good, solid night's sleep is nearly impossible to come by. This leaves you tired all the time, sometimes to such a degree that all you want to do is lie around in bed. Problem is, no one wants to hear this; they look at you in bed all the time and call you a lazy son of a bitch. I practically needed an ejector seat to get me out and moving around. When I managed, I went to the club to work out but there was no greater challenge than the effort to simply leave the bedroom. Post-opioid addiction fatigue is a killer.

One day as I returned from the club Maurine, who was barely speaking to me, handed me the phone and said, "It's your father. Talk to him. Tell him what you've done." I think I would have rather been tortured. This was mean. It was mean and it was lowdown. My father and I'd had a tenuous relationship from my birth, and I disliked the man for how I perceived he'd treated my mother throughout their relationship. But there was *détente* between us because of my high achievements until I flunked my first year of medical school. From that point on, particularly after the passing of my mother and his remarriage, we were almost totally estranged. I did not like the man and I did not feel he cared much for me. I didn't need him and he certainly didn't need me. Now Maurine handed me the phone for what I saw as no practical reason except to punish me some more. Not exactly what I needed right then, but when you screw up like I did, you take your lumps because everyone around you seems to think if they don't punish you, you won't understand you did wrong. Bullshit. I knew I did wrong. I didn't need the world reminding me every second of every day.

When I confronted her, Maurine denied malicious intent, instead saying she did it because he might have some answers for me and might be able to lend me a hand. Hadn't she learned anything about the man after all our years together? I told him my story as succinctly as possible, blaming no one but myself, knowing he wouldn't believe me if I presented it any other way. When I finished, he said gruffly, "Well, you better pull yourself up by your bootstraps. Good luck," and hung up. What I didn't know at the time is it was the best thing he could have done. By not helping me and enabling me, he was helping drive me to my bottom. I didn't know it, I didn't realize it, and at the time, I hated him for it. To this day, I don't know if he did it for the right reasons. Unlike Maurine, I never expected anything positive from the man. Had she not called him, I might never have called him again until I got myself out of the dilemma I was facing. I was beginning to wonder if I would ever climb out of this pit.

Amanda, one of my twins, was newly married and living near Los Angeles. Maurine started spending more and more time visiting her, mostly because she hated talking to me. Two people living under the same roof in silence is uncomfortable as hell. She'd often stay overnight. In a parallel universe, she would have been worried I'd slip and begin using again, but she was too angry with me for that now. If such a thing happened, it simply would have been me lowering myself to her dour expectations.

Chip, our youngest, was in his last year at Georgetown. I sent him to Exeter for a year, and then three-and-a-half years at Georgetown, all on my dime—doctors don't get need-based financial aid. Now the bill arrived for his last semester and I didn't have it. It was mortifying. I wasn't working, Maurine wasn't working, there was no money coming in, and we'd sold off what we could and handed the money to the IRS. The house was for sale but it hadn't sold yet, so we were still living in it, but even once it sold—and I didn't know when that would occur—there wouldn't be enough left over to pay his bill. Chip had to get the money on his own.

Each day felt like things couldn't get any worse. And then they did. Not that Chip didn't know what happened with me and the opioids, but now I had to saddle him personally with the bill for his last semester at an expensive private college. He took out loans for the entire thing, which was a bundle. I could not help him with a dime. His three sisters had gotten a full-ride from me and wanted for nothing except an honest and stable father. Chip would not be as lucky. He had every reason to hate me for that and it killed me inside. I couldn't even attend his graduation. It was partly shame and partly because we could only afford one plane ticket and Maurine chose to go. I stayed in California in case we got a buyer on the house. Never did I feel more left behind. If ever there was a time I wanted to drown myself in a bottle of loneliness it was then, but I proudly remained clean and sober. It was, perhaps, the only thing in which I could take pride.

While Maurine was away, I suffered a massive gastrointestinal bleed. I was so depressed, I wasn't eating. Combine that with my gastric bypass and the aftermath of the opioid and alcohol abuse and I was a physical wreck. I quickly became too dizzy to stand. I was all alone. I had to crawl around the house. I could have called 911, but in my perverse desire to punish myself for my sins, I gutted it out (no pun intended) until I felt well enough to drive myself to the hospital where I'd had my gastric work done. They checked me out and validated that the bleeding had stopped, but they wanted me to come back for thorough and frequent aftercare. I yessed them and went on my way. I had no intention of coming back unless I started bleeding again, nor did I intend on making any positive digestive lifestyle changes. It wasn't as dramatic as suicide, but in the recesses of my mind I didn't give a hot damn whether I lived or died. I might even have been worth more to my family dead than alive.

We finally sold the house, gave Uncle Sam his pound of flesh (to which he was fairly entitled), but were left without enough to even rent a new place. Mortified once more, my daughter Amanda offered us a room in her home, but the whole situation repulsed me. It's not uncommon for your twenty-something kids to find themselves between jobs, needing a place to hang their hat for a few months until they're back up on their feet. But this was her mother and father, their Harvard-trained-doctor father, the man who made her and her siblings want for nothing the entire time they'd been on the planet, and now we couldn't even afford a place to crash. Pathetic. Although Amanda's husband was far from thrilled about it, he, too, was kind enough to allow us to invade his privacy. Perhaps I would have been the same way had it been my own dad who screwed up as I did, but still, it stung. Respect was something I never really felt I had to work hard to get. In fact, I rarely even thought about it. Now I felt ashamed to look my children and their spouses in the eye, wondering what they thought of me and knowing they had every right to disrespect me.

I started looking for employment. The medical community wouldn't touch me, receiving much the same legal advice as my old hospital. As one might imagine, I started with expectations pretty high. I knew who I was and felt I was senior management material—a six-figure-type guy. The world-at-large didn't quite see it that way. My first job was as a bill collector. Once the rubber hit the road, this was too ironic even for me. How the hell could I get rough with someone over the phone when I was being battered from all sides with creditors doing the same to me? I didn't want to hassle those poor folks; I'd hear their sob stories and I wanted to lend them a few bucks out of my own meager pocket. Never before would I have felt this way, but my decline gave me humility and empathy I never knew I had before. I quit the job almost immediately.

I didn't know how to present myself when I applied for jobs. If I said I was a medical doctor, they wondered what the hell I was doing there. If I answered truthfully, they showed me the door. A guy who lost his license for being a junkie was as off-limits as a former felon. If I failed to say I was a doctor, they looked at my resume and had even more questions. I simply could not hit upon a way to spin the whole thing. The truth wasn't working and no lie made any sense. When you present yourself for employment and immediately incite questions about your character and veracity, you're dead meat. There're too many fish in the sea; why would anyone want to get in bed with a problem-child like me? I also learned if you don't have youth, you'd better have specific job experience.

My expectations kept getting lower and lower. I saw an ad for a manager for a new sandwich shop that was opening. Me, a doctor, managing a fast-food joint. But hey, I was in management.

Believe it or not, I didn't fare too badly at first. I swallowed my pride and tried to enjoy the experience. Hard, I know, but I'd grown up in a grocery store so there was a weird sort of sense memory to it all. The kids nicknamed me "Doc," which most doctors hate—me too—but they were the only people referring to me as a doctor so I wore it well. It was better than being called, "Loser." I started to take pride in the work, even in making sandwiches, and daydreamed of maybe owning a franchise or two myself. But who was I kidding? I didn't have the money, and I could have worked there the rest of my life and not been able to put away enough money to buy a place. When I realized that, my brief happiness with the situation began to deteriorate.

By now it had been about seven or eight months since the loss of my license. I'd been clean and sober all that time, but as the days dragged on and I kept putting on that damn sandwich shop hat like a pimply-faced kid, I started to crack. The hat, the job, the nickname, living with my daughter and son-in-law, having only a bedroom to call my own, sharing it with a woman who couldn't stand me and most times wouldn't even talk to me, it was all becoming too much. I started to drink again to dull the pain. No longer was I leaning against a fancy bar at a country club, ordering top-shelf liquor and leaving hundred dollar bills as tips in order to get big pours. Now I was trolling liquor stores looking for the cheapest vodka they carried. It tasted like rubbing alcohol but I didn't care. I was sincerely drinking to get drunk, to ease my pain. I had no other agenda. I was drinking whenever no one was around. I believe people knew; I could tell by the way they looked at me and some little things they'd say, but I didn't really care. If someone found me out, how much lower could I go, and did I care? Where to get the next drink was all that mattered.

Maurine was working, too, which she hadn't done in thirty years, although she's a very intelligent, educated woman. She'd gotten work as a teacher's assistant. It didn't pay well, but it was honest labor and didn't involve slapping cold cuts on bread. And as unhappy as she was, she didn't try to drown her sorrows in liquor. The same could not be said for me.

At the end of the school year, Maurine sought a different position. Aggressive and ambitious, she found it—near San Diego, where we had previously lived. But we didn't have money to afford a place to live. Resourceful as always, she asked an old girlfriend from the Beach and Tennis Club if she could bunk in with her. The girlfriend agreed, but the plan did not include me. The upshot was that Maurine took the job—took it because she knew she had to— and left me. I believe I asked what the long-range plan was and got no real answer. Maurine was so disgusted with me she was calling her own shots and taking care of herself, as well she should have. I was now a drunken anchor weighing her down.

Whereas I took pride in never showing up drunk for work as a doctor, I now drank in order to face having to work in the fast-food business. Drinking after work missed the point entirely. One day I hit my bottom. I showed up drunk, opened the store, and couldn't even stay long enough for the second employee to arrive. Too inebriated to work, I left the place unattended without even leaving a note. Even at a hoagie shop, where the bar is set pretty darn low, this was way over the line.

I ran off, figuring that was the end of that, but the owner actually tracked me down at home and confronted me. I apologized sincerely, admitting to him I was an addict who'd fallen off the wagon. To my surprise, he actually took me back. I hadn't even thought to ask for his forgiveness, but he gave it nonetheless. Chalk it up to altruism or maybe that it was so hard to find help he was willing to put up with an unreliable drunk—take your choice. But he didn't fire me. I came back for a few more weeks, but I repeated the episode over and over again. Not only did I drink on the job, not only did I show up drunk, I'd often either forget to show up at all or show up and leave because I couldn't even function. Even a saint couldn't run a business putting up with such behavior and I was deservedly sacked.

If it were ever a debatable point before, I was now an incorrigible alcoholic. I drank every damn minute I could get my hands on the stuff and I drank every drop until I passed out. Amanda was wonderful to me, all things considered, but her husband was really getting disgusted with me and I don't blame him. He was a young man with a young wife and wanted to have good, happy, independent times, but here I was, the drunken relative who wouldn't leave. A night or two would have been fine, even weeks or months, but it looked like I would be living with them forever, and I'm sure he didn't want to hear it.

Maurine's San Diego school job ended and she wanted to move back to LA. Far more dependable than I, she was earning a small but steady income and set aside enough so we could afford a three-room apartment above a Bikram Yoga studio. Simply defined, Bikram Yoga is "hot" yoga. You do your yoga thing, but you make the room hot as a sweat lodge. Fine for them, but once we moved into the apartment, I came to realize why the place was so affordable. Heat rises. No matter how much we opened the windows or fiddled with the thermostat, our place was almost as hot as the yoga studio. God, we hated it. Funky mold even started growing all over the place. We were living in some crazy hot Petri dish.

Unemployed, I decided to try recovery again, albeit sporadically. I went to some twelve-step meetings and met some fellow addicts. One guy was nice and offered me a job chopping cilantro in his restaurant. This was how far I'd slipped—even in the food service field, I couldn't handle management. I was the guy one step above the floor-sweeper, working for minimum wage. But I took it. In fact, I cried with gratitude when he apologized he couldn't pay me more. God knows no one else wanted me. But I lied, as addicts are wont to do. I may have been going to some meetings, but I was still drinking. Yet I loved this guy so, loved how he had reached out his hand to me when no one else would, that I tried my darndest to at least be sober during the hours I was chopping for him in his restaurant. Outside of that, all bets were off. Still, I only lasted about a month. It had nothing to do with drinking; I simply wasn't good enough! I was an older guy who'd learned to treat his fingers like valuable instruments of healing. Young immigrant workers, happy to have any job at all, were faster than I was and got twice as much done in half as much time. They had to let me go.

Throughout this period, I'd drink whenever I could. If I was sober, it was just for a day or two, or if I simply couldn't cobble together enough pocket change for some rot gut. Even though we had our own place now, Maurine couldn't wait to get away from me. When I'd come home, she'd find every excuse to go visit Amanda or Katie so she wouldn't have to share space with me. Where once I'd been the guy bored with domesticity, now I sat at home staring at walls, spouse-less. My usual routine would be to drink until I passed out so I could spend as much time unconscious as possible, unaware of the passing of days, wasted, wasted days, days full of nothing but pain and hopelessness.

Whatever little buoyancy I had I placed in twelve-step support programs, yet I was expecting the program to do all the work for me. Like the worst of the lot, I'd show up drunk at meetings, which was acceptable so long as you didn't cause a disturbance. But how pathetic! If you don't work the program, the whole thing's a joke. There's no magic bullet. But somehow I thought the meetings could be like my gastric bypass surgery—a quick and easy mechanical way of solving a problem without having to do any work or be at all disciplined. It doesn't work. Hell, with all the resultant health problems I developed, I was living proof that gastric surgery wasn't magical, either.

Losing the kitchen job left me with no reason to wake up in the morning. I even stopped looking for work. I couldn't bring myself to network at the twelve-step meetings because I'd failed at the one shot I'd been given.

Once, in the middle of the day with sun shining all around me, I awoke from a blackout stark naked in my car parked in front of the Petri dish apartment on busy Manhattan Beach Blvd. I still don't know how I got there. There were no clothes in the car. I had to run up the outdoor stairs to gain cover inside. Somehow I managed to do it without being arrested. I can only shudder at what other escapades I engaged in while functionally unconscious.

At what I thought was my lowest point—a point that had become a moving target, I topped it so frequently—I took myself to a charity detox center. No plush Betty Ford Clinic for me. That would have been the way to go back when I was rich Dr. Skip, but now I could only manage a place that would take me for almost nothing, places of which there are frighteningly few. It wasn't completely free; I had to turn to Maurine for a few dollars so they would take me and keep me overnight.

The place was a hellhole. I lasted about seven days. They were so overloaded with clients they had no real bed for me, so I slept on a couch in a storefront window, like a puppy in a pet store. This was not the most therapeutic setting, to say the least, and it made me feel even worse than when I went in. After a few nights they finally had a bed open up, where I had the privilege of sharing barracks-like space with a dozen or so derelicts who were vomiting and passing gas all night long.

Once the facilitators got to know me and my background, they gave me responsibilities they didn't readily give out to most of the rank-and-file addicts, most of whom happened to be lifelong denizens of the outer ridges of society—uneducated and poor, not having had the opportunities I'd had in life. They put me in charge of leading a little field trip where we took a nice, long, healthy walk to a twelve-step meeting a few miles away. On our return, we were thirsty and I took the group to a coffee shop. Bad idea. Whereas most twelve-step meetings could literally get endorsement deals from coffee companies—group members congregate, before and after, around a never-idle coffeemaker and drink like it was the Fountain of Youth—this facility held to the philosophy that caffeine was addictive and thus verboten. I can't really argue with the theory that caffeine *can* be addictive, but still, we'd been walking a long way and we were parched. Not only that, but I'd been given strict instructions and I failed to follow them. Someone reported me and I lost my privileges.

I may have been beaten down beyond all recognition, but I was still irascible. There was a liquor store right next to the detox facility. After getting chewed out, I walked out the door, bought a quart of dirt-cheap vodka, and drank it down. Yell at me for drinking coffee, will ya? I'll show you.

I called Maurine and told her I was coming home. She didn't volunteer to pick me up so I began walking. It was a hell of a long walk—miles. Plus, I was drunk. I stumbled around until dark, then found myself walking through someone's tennis court, which must have looked pretty comfortable to me because I folded my large frame down and went to sleep right there. The next morning I arose, covered in dirt, and continued my trek. I was not welcomed home with open arms. I'd failed again at recovery; I couldn't even manage to stay in an overnight facility, and now I stood before my family dirty, smelly, disgusting to look at, and hung over. What a loser.

When you keep hitting bottom, and then keep moving the bottom lower and lower time after time, it almost becomes like a game. How much lower could I go? I tried to find out. I drowned myself in liquor, attempting to almost give myself alcohol poisoning. Mind you, I still had a resectioned stomach. I was drinking bottle after bottle of hard liquor and my body had been surgically altered to barely accept a small glass of wine. In this condition, I got behind the wheel of a car—God help the poor souls who shared the road with me that day—and drove to LA County USC Medical Center. I walked in and told them I was not suicidal but I was at the end of my rope and didn't know what to do. I found some poor intern and told him the entire tale of "The Rise and Fall of Dr. Skip," ending with the part where here I was, standing before him, drunk as hell, dead broke, crazy, and not knowing what to do next. They helped me by doing exactly what I hoped they would do—putting a seventy-two-hour hold on me in the psych ward. By the time I woke up I had soiled myself and was surrounded by others like me who had done much the same. Some were addicts like me, while others were seriously disturbed.

The doctor who was assigned to me made it evident from his care that he didn't like his job, didn't like me, and didn't want to be there. He had to get a baseline of medical data from me, as is done with all patients. He touched his stethoscope to my chest for less than the length of the heartbeat and pulled it away as if he didn't want to soil it. I stared at him and said, "What did you hear? You weren't there long enough to hear a goddamn thing and you know it. I know you don't like me, but you have an obligation to your craft to do your job right. You don't have to like me or approve of me, but you have to still be a doctor." He didn't like that one bit, but it got me agitated enough that I almost started to feel like my old self. I was back in a hospital and I was exposing a young resident for not doing his job and for not caring. I was me again, after a fashion—sense memory, just like when I was working around food. It brought me back to a better place, a better me.

They tried to release me, but had to find a family member to pick me up. They called Katie, who told them "No way! Keep him there; he's a danger." They shipped me over to a mental hospital, which kept me another six or seven days. Katie wasn't being hateful; she just knew my MO. She knew, even when impaired, I could talk my way out of just about anything, and she figured I'd tried to talk my way out of being hospitalized and she wasn't going to be a part of it. My first-born, with her big, blueberry eyes, had been so kind to me at my worst and most disgusting moments. I know she was afraid for me and did the right thing.

The law in California is after five or six days an officer of the court comes in and the medical facility has to present its case for holding you for more than a week. It's a sort of legal hearing to make sure people aren't being falsely imprisoned. By this time I'd had more than enough time to be detoxed. Now the only question was whether I was certifiably insane. I wasn't, nor did I wish to attempt to prove I was. I'd become bored with the whole place and was even pretending to be a doctor again, making sure everyone knew exactly what my educational pedigree was and piping up with suggestions and answering questions that were in no way directed toward me. Some folks found me helpful, while to others I was probably a pain in the ass. Either way, I wasn't crazy and I was not a true danger to myself or others, in the classic definition of the phrase. Katie and Amanda broke down and came by to pick me up and bring me home. These are not demonstrative women, and yet they walked in holding hands, trying to brace one another and give one another strength. I noticed the fear in their eyes as I walked toward them. I was not all right.

This was still not the end of my drinking. For the next month or two I was every bit the incorrigible addict. I drank as much as I could get my hands on and I drank to get drunk and pass out. I stole from Maurine and I stole from my kids. I had no shame whatsoever. If I saw a buck, I'd grab it and take it to the liquor store. I'd have half a bottle in my gullet before I'd even reach home. I didn't care. My two-year sentence was becoming as interminable as if I were in a maximum-security prison with the worst killers and rapists in the world. The only thing was, I was doing it all to myself. Yes, the world was beating me down, but for every unfair slap I'd take, I'd bring on a million more slaps I richly deserved. It was like the beaten man who refuses to cry "uncle" in a street fight. Do you give up? No. Give up now? No. Just keep hitting me; keep hitting me, world. I don't know whether I was trying to prove I could take it or whether it was some form of oblique suicide, goading fate into helping me die.

Drinking right in front of Maurine was too much for her to bear. She'd give me hell, which I richly deserved, but I couldn't help myself and I didn't want to put up with her bitching and yelling. I had to find sanctuary for myself and my liquor. The roof. The damn apartment was always so hot because of the yoga studio below that sitting out on the roof was a way to keep cool. It also became a place to hide from my wife. I'd go up there with a bottle or two and drink until I passed out. How I managed not to kill myself while up there, God only knows. The thought of suicide passed through my mind more than once, but a dramatic leap from the roof wasn't something I could motivate myself to do. Maybe it was fear, maybe it was morality, maybe it was the cognizance that since at its highest point it was only three stories off the ground, I wasn't high enough to guarantee death from the fall and I might simply hurt or cripple myself, which would make me even more miserable than I already was. The mode I was in was death by habit, suicide by personal neglect. I was like a 500-pound man eating bacon burgers morning, noon, and night. I knew exactly what I was doing. It was simply more pleasurable than putting a bullet in my head.

Sometimes I didn't even bother coming home in order to escape Maurine and the heat by heading for the roof. Often on the way to the roof I'd have to pass Maurine, which gave her ample opportunity to chew me out for being a degenerate drunk. Who needs that? So, many nights instead of coming home from the liquor store, I'd sleep wherever I could—in a car, in an alleyway, on the beach. I was choosing to present myself to the world as not only an addict, but a homeless one, too.

December 1, 2000. I was on the roof and still had half a bottle to go. People talk about moments of clarity. This was mine. I asked myself the rhetorical: *What am I doing up here?* When you get used to passing out, you pass out for shorter and shorter periods of time. You get no rest. It seemed like I was only away from my problems for minutes. I looked like a filthy bastard, I felt like a filthy bastard, I smelled like a filthy bastard. I'd become a decrepit, degenerate bum. I wasn't this way before. I wasn't even this bad when I started doing the opioids. Hell, I wasn't this bad when I got *caught* doing the opioids. I'd made a conscious choice to turn myself into the worst caricature of an addicted loser I could ever imagine. Why? Why was I doing this? What was the long-range plan, the end game, the goal? What sign was I looking for?

Something flipped in my brain. I was not forgiving myself or denying to myself that I was an addict. But I wasn't *this* kind of addict. This was an outright joke, a farce I was playing upon myself. All my life I'd drink, I'd stop; I'd perform well. The idea I was incorrigible was a lie. It was a costume I'd decided to wear for some crazy reason. Just as I'd given up drinking before, I could do it again. I could do it for as long as I chose. That was how it was when I played football. My future was mine. If I wanted to be a social drinker again, I felt I could. Or if I wanted to abstain completely, I could do that as well. It felt no different from when I first stepped into Boston College High or Harvard. I was confused, afraid, and then it hit me: *I'm not* like *those alcoholics; I'm one of them.* My life changed at that moment. *I can do this.* A flash of insight or a spiritual awakening? I'm not sure which it was, but it started me on the road back. Although I tend to believe it was my Higher Power, I leave that to those who are more spiritually certain.

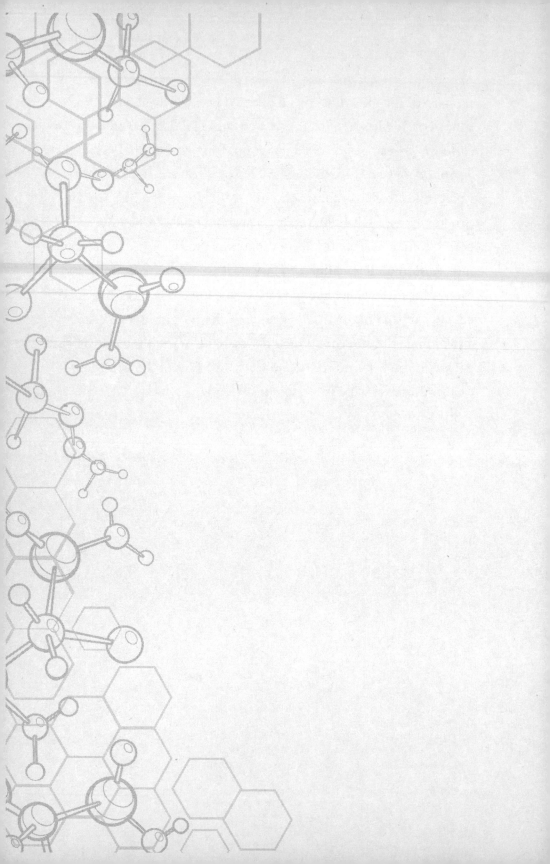

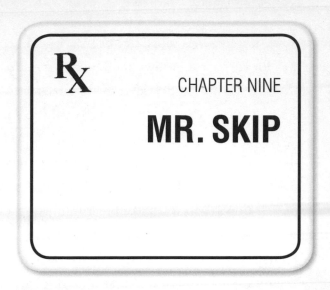

CHAPTER NINE

MR. SKIP

I climbed down from the roof. I left my last bottle, which was not yet empty, on the roof of the apartment above the yoga studio and climbed back into our place. I made no loud pronouncements; I just never drank again. I quietly told Maurine I was through with drinking. She didn't believe me and I didn't blame her. I started going to meetings, getting support, and instead of just talking about it, I lived it. "One day at a time," is a tired cliché, but for me, it was about the peace, solitude, and simplicity of the statement. Only one day. No bigger commitment than that. One day. Shut your damn big mouth, put your head down and work, and just try to not screw up for one twenty-four-hour period. That's all. Maurine no longer believed in me and that was okay. I'd just turn it around one day at a time.

I started a new ritual in our marriage. Every day, I would make a point to walk up to her and kiss her. It wasn't about the affection. It was a usually a quick kiss on her cheek or neck, but what I really wanted was for her to smell me. For all the days of my heaviest addiction, I would avoid coming too close to her. Get too close and she would be able to smell the liquor on me. By kissing her every day, I was wordlessly telling her, "See, I don't smell. No liquor on me." I didn't even smell like breath mints or toothpaste—the sorts of things people try in order to mask the booze. No, I was clean. At first, she would resist me. I disgusted her. I knew that, knew it even more once I got into recovery. But I loved her, and as long as we were still under the same roof, I hoped somewhere deep in her heart she loved me, too. She was just damn angry and disappointed in me and she had a right to those feelings. But each day, even if she tried running or pushing away, I managed to plant a kiss on her. Eventually, it became easier. Finally, she started to reciprocate. If I kept making proclamations, as I had over the years, she would have shot me down. Instead, I said nothing but a kiss. The kiss was proof I was telling the truth.

I found an ad for a job in a clinic dealing with schizophrenia and substance abuse. A doctor by the name of John ran the operation. He needed helpers to pick up and transport people with mental health issues. I got hired as an assistant counselor, although there was no real counseling involved on my part, nor was I trained in counseling. I was basically an entry-level healthcare assistant, hired to take mentally incapacitated people to outings such as the zoo or the beach. A glorified babysitter.

I hated the job. It was like being a hospital orderly. My, how the mighty had fallen. But as luck would have it, before I was tempted to drink my way out of that job as well, a guy in middle management quit and a spot opened up. Everyone who worked with me knew I was far, far, far overqualified for what I was doing, so they offered to move me up, thank God. Not only was the new position a step up, it was a massive rise monetarily, paying nearly three times the entry-level wage.

Again, I threw myself into a job, but this time I found a little more staying power, since it was the first job I'd had since being stripped of my license that sort of reminded me of what I had once been—a physician and medical administrator. I whipped the place into shape much as I had numerous emergency rooms under my care. I had something in which to take pride once more. It was a good feeling.

I managed to take my earnings, combine them with Maurine's, and we got a slightly better apartment in Redondo Beach, one without a hot yoga studio below us. Our lot was improving ever so slightly. My children and their spouses were less bitter and resentful toward us because we were finally carrying most of our own load. When Maurine would visit them it was to help rather than to impose upon them. Even I began visiting again, less ashamed of myself.

There is a federal Office of the Inspector General for the Department of Health. A law came down stating that when a person loses his or her medical license, his or her Medicare number is taken away. Initially, this was interpreted as placing the former physician's name on a Medicare fraud list, which was fine because if you don't have a license, you certainly shouldn't be sending new bills to Medicare as a provider. Getting off that blacklist was a bureaucratic pain in the ass, but it was doable. But by the time I lost my license, the mandate of the law expanded. Suddenly, you could not even be

an *employee* of someone who accepted Medicare if your name was
on that list of defrocked medical professionals. And it wasn't limited
to physicians. It covered nurses, therapists, you name it. It mattered
not that I wasn't the owner or operator. I was merely an employee,
but I was on the list of untouchables. They went to Dr. John and
told him he had twenty-four hours to can me.

I had done nothing newly wrong. This was all from my prior
incident writing Vicodin scripts to myself. Outside of that, all
my horrible, self-destructive, alcoholic behavior had somehow
managed to not turn up on their radar. I could have been an angel,
not imbibing anything stronger than a glass of milk and this still
would have come down upon my head. I felt it was unfair. I was
in no position now to do anything illegal as a doctor, so why did
they have to take away my ability to work for someone else in a
nonmedical capacity? I didn't understand their thinking at all. It was
like losing your driver's license and being told that disqualified you
from getting a job working from home. No linkage whatsoever.

Dr. John was as decent as possible about it. He gave me a
month's severance pay, which he didn't have to do, and luckily I'd
lasted at that job long enough to apply for unemployment. By then
I'd been in recovery for over a year. I felt healthy and my mind was
clear. This was a setback, but I was well on my way to better things,
so I managed a stiff upper lip and did not use this as an excuse to
backslide to my wicked ways.

My two-year sentence as a banished doctor was coming to an
end. I had gotten myself through those two years by telling myself
once that time was up I'd reapply, get my license back, and this hell
would be over. Truth was, they had only said after two years I was
allowed to reapply. That's a hell of a big difference than saying after

two years I would be handed my life back. Anyone is *allowed* to apply to Harvard; it doesn't mean they all get in.

I began my reinstatement procedure with some trepidation. Was I sober? "Yes." I was finessing the query. Since all they'd busted me for was opioids, I limited my answer, in my own mind, to that issue alone. Had I been opioid-free since they took my license? Why yes. If they had asked me specifically about drinking I might have had to tell the truth, but they failed to do so and thus I was less than forthcoming. Besides, I was sober on the day they asked.

Leading up to any formal reinstatement hearing was a pronouncement that I was still subject to criminal proceedings. This was a completely separate issue in a way, although the fruits of this investigation would factor into whether the medical board would allow me back. It struck me as odd at first, that there would be such a lapse of time between my meeting with the medical board and having to meet with the distict attorney's office, but the medical board felt it had a more acute situation to deal with, while the DA felt quite the opposite—that I was primarily accused of a victimless crime and not an immediate danger to anyone but myself, so their office dragged its heels and allowed time to pass before getting around to me.

I was scared out of my wits. Appearing in front of administrative types is not extremely intimidating. Appearing before people with the power to put you behind bars is a different story entirely. The San Diego District Attorney showed my lawyer that the police had been following me and tracing my paper trail of prescriptions from pharmacy to pharmacy. They showed us the testimony from the nurses I'd involved. That part hurt, since I'd gotten many of them in trouble and they didn't deserve that. I always treated nurses well and these nurses, even though I'd damaged their careers, said some awfully nice things about me in their affidavits. It was rather apparent they would never have stuck their necks out in the first place for a doctor they thought was a jerk. They likely would have gotten him busted long before the walls came crashing down on them. None of those nurses did anything to "narc me out." Only when they were forced to testify against me did they offer the truth. I'll never forget their loyalty to me as a person. Perhaps they would have been doing me a bigger favor had they not helped me, but still, I knew they were good people and I knew they thought I was a good person, which only made me feel more horrible for what I had done.

We were about to make a plea bargain when the DA postulated it was impossible I could have written all those Vicodin prescriptions to myself; that I had to have been selling drugs to others. As I had before when I faced the medical board, I told them I crawled around on the floor chasing stray pills, so desperate was I for my high. I would not have shared one single pill with someone else for all the money in the world.

For once I lucked out, getting a kind and understanding criminal judge who gave me three years probation, which he eventually knocked down to eighteen months because of my recovery.

With this part of the ordeal behind me, I made my first foray before the medical board. Not so fast, they said. Even though I was in recovery now, even though I had a good record of employment with Dr. John—who was kind enough to appear on my behalf and vouch for my good behavior—they wanted more time. "More time for what?" I asked. More recovery. More documentation of good behavior. Just more of everything. I felt this was arbitrary and it was. Still, all they'd promised me was the *opportunity* to apply for reinstatement. From there, they were on their own. They felt they could pretty much do with me as they liked, so long as it did not appear overly capricious or biased based on race, religion, etc. From then on I kept a log of all my relevant activities and sent it to them once a month. They said they wanted me to take a proficiency test. Fine. I'll take any test you want to throw at me. I felt confident in my medical knowledge. Time kept moving along. By now it was three-and-a-half years since my loss of license.

The test was allegedly for general medical knowledge. No problem. It was to be an oral exam. I went in and the proctors were two emergency-medicine specialists. Great! My specialty. It was also readily apparent I was older and had logged more ER hours than both of these guys. What could they hit me with that I didn't already know?

New stuff. While I answered everything correctly, they would follow up with, "But is that the newest medication for treating X, Y, and Z?" Newest? How new? It was a trick, a trap. My answers weren't wrong, but pharmacology keeps moving on, new drugs coming on the market every day. What was popular four years ago still worked, but it wasn't the most popular "new" medicine now. Consider Prozac. It was the first generation of antidepressant. Today, much of its market share is dwarfed by newer drugs. But does Prozac still work? Yes, and some patients are still on it. So if I were asked what to prescribe for depression, answering, "Prozac" would not be an incorrect answer. But it wouldn't be the answer they wanted and they told me so.

What complicated this even more was that the board had already informed me that returning to emergency medicine was off the table, at least for the time being. I'd have to find another specialty where I'd have more supervision and it would be harder for me to swipe drugs or write scripts by myself. Yet here I was, being tested by ER physicians. What's up with that?

My overall test grade was well above passing, but because I told them I did not know of all the very latest drugs on the market, they recommended I brush up on this and be supervised and monitored to make sure I did. I had no real problem with that. Any doctor who took time off would do the same thing voluntarily, and I certainly would have of my own volition. I got a letter from the testing supervisor saying I'd passed my test, with that little proviso.

Some bureaucrat called me up and told me I'd failed. I told her she was wrong; I had the document in my hand saying I'd passed. No, she said, I'd failed. This went back and forth like "Who's on first?" I bitched and complained but I was out of resources and had no one I could call upon who could help me. But the bottom line remained the same: the board's decision—and the decision of the state of California—was theirs and theirs alone and unless I could prove some sort of traditionally recognized legal bias, they could do most anything to me they wanted.

At the end of my criminal probation, I went back before the administrative judge. Again, I marched people before him to testify on my behalf. Again I was asked about the aftercare for my addiction and again my performance was true. Since that December night on the roof of that crummy, hot apartment, I had not drunk a drop. He commended me and wrote a letter to the medical board, recommended my license be reinstated. The board ignored him. Instead, they wanted another hearing.

I had dealt with bureaucracy all my life, particularly so being a medical professional. Yet I had never seen anything like this. There was the criminal justice system—I did all they required of me and they seemed satisfied I had paid my debt to society. Then there was the medical board, filled mostly with my peers. But overseeing the medical board were California civil servants—people from Consumer Affairs and such. This third branch of confusion and bluster seemed particularly peeved with me. Now *they* assigned a staffer to whom I was to report. This person was not a doctor. He had just come over from the penal system. I was his first doctor. He was used to dealing with people in maximum-security prisons. Maybe he hated all doctors; I don't know. But he was like the clichéd tough prison guard in some bad movie. His thing was to never, ever refer to me as "Doctor." Not that I insisted on it, but after half a lifetime of being called by that title, I got kind of used to it. Not this guy. He said, "From now on you're to be called 'Mr. Sviokla.' You've lost your right to that other title." No one else in the system was acting so gruff, but this guy must have been slapped damn hard by the doctor who delivered him because he was taking it out on me now. It's surprising how often such a thing would come up. I was "Dr. Sviokla" or "Dr. Skip." That's my name. Everyone around me called me that.

Apparently, this guy's attitude became infectious. I had another of my many hearings—it seemed I was now having them on a regular basis, since I refused to give up my fight to get my license back—and some new guy from the state attorney general's office came to give a report and recommendation. This guy, too, made a big point of referring to me over and over again as "Mr. Sviokla." But it wasn't just that. It was the tone; it was the words describing me. This AG, like the Consumer Affairs guy, *hated* me. I wasn't used to being hated. Maybe if I had gotten drunk and killed his mother, then I would have understood the fury. And yes, I know quite well I *could* have done such a thing. But I didn't. Not only that, but as I've said a hundred times, I never worked on patients while impaired. But this was personal to them. This guy and the other didn't just call me "Mister Sviokla"; they hissed it.

During this particular hearing, one of the men on the board, an older doctor, finally had enough. He raised his hand to quiet the attorney and said, "Listen. This man went to a reputable college, the best medical school in the country, and you have absolutely no right not to call him 'doctor.' You can fight against him getting a license in this state, but why are you insulting him? He's here, he's contrite; he's paid a hefty penalty. Why are you so down on him? Did you even know this man before you met him here today? Had you even laid eyes on him before? Just give us the facts of the case, unenhanced by your own vitriol, and trust us to do our job."

Despite this one man's humanity and compassion, I saw the handwriting on the wall. For everything I did, for every hearing I went to, every monitoring I agreed to, every additional passage of time, the goalposts kept getting moved further and further from sight. Why had I bothered getting into recovery? What was the point? California had decided to make an example of me. Who needs that? Still, what was my next move? And at what point would this make me say, "Screw it all," and go back to drinking?

R~X~ CHAPTER TEN

ON THE **ROAD** TO **RHODE** ISLAND

When I first got into recovery—when it really took—I threw myself into it with a passion heretofore unknown to me. Many sources recommend going to ninety meetings in your first ninety days. I must have gone to 250. I was going to two or three meetings a day, every day. I bonded with all sorts of people in recovery. One meeting I loved to attend was held in the home of a guy from the rock-and-roll scene, which attracted a lot of musicians and artistic types. It might sound strange, but recovery can be as interesting as you make it. Instead of hanging out in drugged out, drunken LA rock clubs, I was getting my fill of elbow-rubbing with rockers and talking about the music I loved in the safe and sober confines of recovery. Another guy I met there owned a motorcycle shop and hung out with a lot of bikers. He became a good friend. I grew up in a working-class town but maybe I lost some of that grit somewhere along the way. When I went to meetings with Viet Nam vets, amputees, street people, dishwashers with little to no education, I got things out of the process I did not get when I went to a meeting in someone's mansion. There was a fluidity to their stories. They didn't make up excuses. There was no spin. They took more personal responsibility for what they did. Some other meetings would devolve into discussions about everything *but* recovery— people complaining about what a hassle addiction was and how it was causing them to miss their island vacations and whatnot. I was really enjoying the wide range of people I was meeting. That would eventually have a serious impact not only on my path of recovery, but also in my overall future.

On a certain level, being a good liar can be a major asset to being a success in this world. The rougher trade I was spending time with weren't as good at lying, which made them more transparent. The exception was the opioid addicts. When you're lying constantly simply in order to get your high—since opioids are illegal—you become incredibly good at it. Opioid addicts can spin incredible stories with vivid detail, and good lies usually have lot of detail. A lot of that is the effect of opioids on the brain; you can see the frantic chaos of it on a PET scan. It's similar to what occurs in severely impaired long-term alcoholics due to their thiamine deficiency. The lies become less and less conscious and more of a break with reality. The more time I spent in these meetings with different sorts of addicts—some of them really hardcore, some of them in greater denial than others, some of them more forthcoming—the more I learned about myself and my own addiction. The meetings became an education for me, not just as an addict, but as a physician as well. I became a better listener and I quickly learned who was telling the truth and who wasn't.

I also came to develop healthy skepticism toward certain aspects of certain recovery groups and programs. In the end, it's all about what works for you. I went to a ton of meetings initially, but then backed off somewhat. Some will tell you if you do that, you'll drift back into using. Maybe yes, but not exclusively. Recovery is not a one-size-fits-all thing, which again was a lesson worth learning. Also, not all groups are the same. I learned finding the group that felt right was incredibly important, and if something doesn't feel right, don't feel guilty about admitting it and moving on. Some were too cult-like for my tastes, with sponsees asking their sponsors when they should go to the bathroom, whom they should date, what they should eat, etc. To me, that was codependent, and if I was anything, it wasn't that. I recall one meeting that particularly turned me off run by, ironically, a doctor in recovery. Nonetheless, he had a helluva reputation in the recovery community and I thought, perhaps, he could help me. I introduced myself to him afterward and upon learning I, too, was a doctor, he invited Maurine and me to join him and his wife for a private get-together. I hoped this could be a turning point for me, since this occurred very early on in my attempts at recovery, prior to my moment of clarity on the hot apartment roof.

I took the opportunity to ask him tons of questions, but what I got in return I found utterly unsatisfying. Homilies. Bumper stickers. Sure, we all know a cliché becomes popular because there's usually a significant truth behind it, but still, I was a drowning man grasping for anything to hold onto. Don't do a private meeting with me just so you can tell me word-for-word what I can read in a thousand books. When we parted, I was blue. Maurine, who tended more often than not to side against me during this tumultuous period, said, "Did you notice how dead his eyes looked?" That jolted me. She summed up what I was thinking. This guy had been in the addiction recovery scene so long he no longer looked at people as individuals. I don't even know if he was enjoying life. He'd become a human cliché machine, and Maurine and I, despite being neophytes, saw right through it. It didn't make him a bad guy, but it taught me there was more to recovery than rote memorization. Thank God I found better meetings as time progressed. They helped me get through the frustrating times.

My daughter, Amanda, and her husband moved to Redondo Beach, where Maurine and I were renting an apartment. Soon thereafter, she blessed us with our first grandchild, Liam. With addiction, people use the phrase, "clean slate" a lot. It's a thing we all wish we had, yet realize we'll never truly possess. The exception is with little babies. Sure, someday Liam might hear about how sick his grandfather once was, but that would only happen after we'd had opportunity to bond. And bond we did. Liam became the greatest joy of my life. I would eventually have six other grandchildren who would also fill my heart with joy, but Liam, being the first, paved the way for the rest. Our love for one another is boundless. He always smiled for me, but by the time he was able to stand up, his special affection for me was apparent to all. While all my kids and their spouses slowly warmed to my newfound recovery—some slower than others—there was little Liam, an explosion of unlimited enthusiasm whenever he saw me coming. I needed that. I needed that badly. It got to a point where I'd practically ignore everyone else and focus all my attention on Liam. This was totally unlike me. I like kids, but I was never a big "kid" person, particularly when they are so small. Let's face it; they don't have a lot of fascinating opinions on the events of the day. What do they do? Eat, sleep, play, and cry.

When I pulled up to his house, Liam would do pirouettes for me; that's how excited he'd get. I was Santa Claus, Ronald McDonald, and the Easter Bunny all rolled up in one. What he may never know is how I truly needed someone, anyone, to feel that way about me right about then. And that's why God made Liam.

My unemployment benefits were running out and California seemed unrelenting to me and my situation. As much as we both loved being around little Liam, Maurine came up with the idea that maybe I would be treated more fairly in some other state. Problem was, neither of us was keen on playing pin-the-tale-on-the-donkey with a US map and ending up somewhere neither of us had any ties or connections. Life can be pretty lonely as it is. That made New England the logical choice. While we'd both come from Massachusetts, we didn't feel quite that limited, and so Maurine started scouting possibilities throughout that general area. It's not uncommon for addicts to want to pick up and move far away in search of that ever-elusive clean slate, but this was more than that. What else can you do when you've been professionally blacklisted?

She found Dr. David Lewis from Brown University in Providence, RI and began a correspondence. Dr. Lewis had never been an addict himself, but he'd been seriously involved in addiction medicine ever since he graduated from my old alma mater, Harvard Medical School. One day she turned to me and told me she'd like me to call him. I scoffed. Why would this guy give me the time of day? But she assured me he would take my call.

Dr. Lewis did not disappoint. He listened to my entire tale of woe and at its conclusion suggested I come to Rhode Island, where he would advocate for me if everything I'd said was true. This felt like the dawning of a new day, like someone had opened the door of a fetid room I was in and let the bugs crawl out.

Maurine found a job an hour away from Providence, in Marshfield, Massachusetts of all places, as a French teacher. Marshfield was where my loving father lived with his second wife. Maurine went east for an interview and was hired. Now we had to find a place to live. The rift between my father and me still had not penetrated Maurine's consciousness, as she suggested I call him to ask if he'd help us find (and possibly help pay for) housing. I did the next best thing, calling on my brother, Francis. Francis was much more accommodating than my father ever could be. He owned a little summer shack on the marshes of Green Harbor, right down the road from Marshfield. The place didn't even have heat, but it was four walls and a roof and the price was right—free.

I said my good-byes to Amanda and Liam, which broke my heart. My daughter Katie was also living nearby at this time as well. Katie had been extremely kind to me. Amanda and Katie had borne the brunt of my worst days. Nicole and Chip, once he graduated from Georgetown, were on the east coast and somewhat insulated from the carnage. They knew what was going on, but they didn't have to see it up close except on holidays. I feel sorry for the kids, as I feel sorry for Maurine. There's a strange dynamic that occurs when one parent is severely addicted. Your kids love you no matter what, even if they don't always say so or act it. Because of that, the more disgusting you get, the more afraid they are that they may have some part in it, that they can make it worse if they do or say the wrong thing. This is ridiculous, but they see themselves as human starter pistols, which is a terrible burden to bear. Because of this, they instead confront the healthy parent—in our case, Maurine. Things they wanted to say to me, they said to her. As if her life couldn't get any worse. Me, they'd avoid because they abhorred my behavior so much. They also held her responsible for my behavior. "Why can't you control him?" That's wrong, too—not just with me, but with any addict.

Maurine returned and we had a garage sale and sold off everything we could from the Redondo apartment and got on a plane bound for Providence. We arrived in summer, so the conditions in the shack were not so bad, but as fall began, things got more frantic, as Maurine had a low-paying job and I had none. When I first arrived, I called up Dr. Lewis and we met face-to-face for the first time. Meanwhile, I started the process of reactivating my Rhode Island medical license, which I'd once possessed but had let lapse. I was forthright with the Rhode Island board, telling them every single detail of my escapades in California. They asked me to immediately be evaluated by a psychiatrist so they could get an unbiased opinion of my mental stability. Addiction is a disease, and in the medical community it is categorized as a disease of the mind.

They recommended Dr. Jon Grant, who was doing a year at Butler Hospital in Providence and whom I came to respect immensely. He evaluated me and said I had some narcissistic qualities (unsurprising to me and most who knew me), but I didn't have a full-blown personality disorder. The bottom line, though, was he gave me the green light to work again as a physician. By now I hadn't drunk a drop in years, and drug abuse was completely off the table.

Dr. Howard Baden, who helped get me into Harvard Medical School, was far more intelligent than I could ever aspire to be. It wasn't until I met Jon Grant many years later that I found someone else I was sincerely in awe of intellectually. Those two operate on a much higher plane. For once, it had nothing to do with wealth or fame. They are geniuses who humble me in a healthy way.

The Rhode Island Medical Board was pretty straightforward with me, which was all I asked. They said based on where I stood and what price I had already paid in California, their recommendation was that I be given back my license under the strict terms of a five-year contract. For five years I would have certain restrictions and oversights, although I would once again be a full-fledged doctor—no more "Mr. Skip" for me. I had to go to a meeting once a month and submit to random drug screenings— at least eight a month for the first year and then slightly fewer in subsequent years. I had to attend some type of twelve-step program with relative regularity and I had to see a counselor.

The counselor they assigned me was a licensed clinic social worker with a master's degree. Don't ask me why, but in the face of all I'd been through, this last request was the one that pissed me off the most. I went to see the guy and told him straight off I was insulted I was mandated to see him. He wasn't even a doctor. What the hell did he know?

Years and years later, I still see him each and every week. He's a brilliant man and he sees clearly for me when I can't. He's a straight-shooter and I tell him the truth. Apparently, I needed someone like that in my life, and the more time I spent with him, the more I realized it. All the things I'd accomplished early in my life had built me up for the fall I had to take. I was damaged, yet I lacked the humility to fully realize it and address my issues.

This was all fine and good, but I was still without a job and winter was coming. Hell, even fall can get damn cold in New England. We bought as many space heaters as we could afford and as many as the ancient electrical system of that little cabin could handle but it wasn't enough. It was like living in a cave. First the steambath above the yoga studio and now this. God was getting me, but good.

We gathered our pennies together and managed to rent a house in Marshfield, not far from my father's beautiful four-bedroom house on the water—in which he only uses one of those bedrooms. But I never asked for his help this time. I was too resentful. I'd been kicked and kicked far too much. I deserved most of those kicks, but still, I wasn't a masochist. Yet it galled me that I could actually see his house from mine. What a strange feeling that was. We were close enough to touch and yet never were we further apart.

Dr. Grant, the psychiatrist assigned to evaluate me, led the Rhode Island Medical Society doctors-only recovery group once a week, which I attended and loved. I came to love Rhode Island and the people I was dealing with there. So many of them—Dr. Grant, Dr. Lewis, and many others—were salt-of-the-earth people who looked beyond punishment and the need to "send a message" to addicts that they'd done something bad to themselves and potentially to others. It made me recall one of the first recovery meetings I'd tried many years before in California. I had decided to get up and give my anonymous testimony. Right in the middle of my tale, where I mentioned a drinking binge I had gone on with another nameless doctor, some woman got up and heckled me. Heckled me! How dare I, a doctor, be a user? Luckily for me, the crowd booed her and she left, but I was scarred by the experience and didn't go to another meeting for years thereafter. Apparently it was fine for her and everyone else in the room to be an addict; it simply wasn't tolerable that a doctor was, too. Now I was in a meeting with nothing but doctors, and despite the more positive experiences I'd had in group recovery in the ensuing years, this relaxed me and opened me up even more since I knew we all had something in common. It was a no-heckle zone.

Not that anyone has it easy, but doctors have a uniquely difficult time in recovery. First, there's the "God complex" thing. We're in a field where people die in our arms and we're supposed to step away and go on to the next patient—shake it off. The only way you can do that is by leaving certain feelings behind, like any shades of guilt or responsibility. If you're working on that next patient while thinking about the last, "Did I do something wrong? Was it my fault? Is there something I could have done differently?" you can't function. You'll kill the new patient. So already, we've got a developed personality pattern of omnipotence. But how do the omnipotent ask for help? How do they admit defeat? How do they admit something is stronger than they are? It's hard.

Dr. Lewis advised me to meet with another addiction medicine specialist. It wasn't for treatment; hell, I was getting all sorts of treatment whether I wanted it or not. I was looking for a damn job. He sat me down with a few of his medical colleagues and asked me what I wanted to do with my life. I told him I doubted emergency-room medicine would be a good fit for me going forward. California had singled that out as a potential trouble spot for a guy like me, and Rhode Island was taking a lot of its cues from California. Perhaps I could have fought that point and won, but I didn't really have the fight in me. It wasn't the most important thing. Hell, I still dreamed of being a surgeon, except that wasn't happening, either. Surgery had passed me by just as professional football had. The time had come and gone.

When California put the kibosh on ER medicine, I started to daydream of what I would do instead. Recovery had a profound effect on me. I'd met a lot of great doctors in addiction medicine. A few jerks, too, but seeing both ends of the spectrum was good for me. On one hand, it showed me how this specialty could open up wonderful possibilities for compassionate care. On the other, it showed me some guys did it well, while others sucked at it and I could bring a better perspective to the job than they. I'd spent most of my life thinking of myself. Sure, I took care of patients, but that was my job and I wanted to do my job well. The concept of truly "giving back" had not really been in my vernacular. That was the biggest change that occurred because of my addiction and recovery. Now I wanted to give something back to the world without asking for anything in return.

When I cut my hand, killing off my surgical career, I hadn't realized how God had given me a lucky break as a sort of consolation prize. Emergency medicine was a new and burgeoning specialty. I initially took to it for all the wrong reasons and my head was in a terrible, depressed place, but in the end it allowed me to prosper. Now that ER medicine appeared off-limits to me, my interest in addiction medicine coincided with a similar set of circumstances. For decades, even centuries, addiction was treated shabbily in the medical, legal, and social communities. Addicts were weak, self-destructive people who chose to slowly commit suicide. *To hell with them all.* When they got bad enough, you threw them in jail or in a mental institution so they wouldn't harm others. Today though, things were changing. Miracle drugs like Suboxone, for opioid addiction, as well as other treatments were coming onto the market. Enlightenment was occurring and I was in the right place at the right time so I could really help people.

I also felt addiction medicine would be a safe haven for me as a recovering addict. I'd had one bad experience already in California when I tried going into recovery and had not yet lost my license. Everyone fears losing his or her anonymity, but we doctors are among the most paranoid of the bunch. A nurse who was moved to my department came up to me and said, "I hear you're coming to our meetings now and so-and-so is your new sponsor. That's great! I'll so enjoy working with you and seeing you at meetings." My head exploded. I was still an ER doctor. What this nurse did was totally wrong no matter what we both did for a living, and I scolded her and my sponsor about it. But as we go through life, we try to learn from our mistakes. I'd already tried never going into group recovery again, but that hadn't worked very well. One constructive take-away from this little drama was if I was ever outed again, better that I be around addicts, treating them as a fellow addict, than were I to be in some other area of medicine. You can never fear the skeletons in your closet if you bring them out yourself.

The addiction-medicine specialist I had met with mulled it over and decided to give me a chance. I came to learn he found his calling in addiction medicine because he had lost his brother to a drunk driver. There *but for the grace of God go I*. I began doing his patient intakes, which is medical grunt work but it felt good to be back in the game. It was also a particularly good place for me. I was one of the first faces addicts would see. I would be one of the first people to whom they'd tell their story. Me, a recovering addict myself. I imagine even the expressions on my face as they told their stories differed from that of someone who had never walked in their shoes. I was good at this. Not that I was an expert yet. I had a lot yet to learn, but I took a unique and personal interest in that schooling. In learning how to treat others, I was coming to learn more about myself. What a motivator!

I started off making less than most kids are paid in entry-level jobs but still, it felt invigorating. I was a doctor again. Might not have been paid like a doctor, but it was better than chopping cilantro. Once you added my salary to Maurine's, we were suddenly solid, working-class people. It was a hell of a comedown from my years making half a million per, but to us, it felt like we'd hit the lottery. "Grateful" would be the best way of describing it.

Each day I learned more and more. I joined the American Society of Addiction Medicine and became certified. I enjoyed studying the field. I thrived on it. There was so much going on of which I was unaware. Again, the timing was such that I felt I came to this area of medicine at an exciting and heady point in its development. I went to the Rhode Island Medical Board and they helped me get my DEA certification back, allowing me to write prescriptions. I was still under contract, but the shackles were coming off ever so gradually. With each baby step, I was positioning myself to be more of a full-fledged, independent doctor as I once had been. Even though I was working in the medical field once more, the process was to treat me like a little kid—first a tricycle, then a two-wheeler with training wheels, and if I was good, eventually a two-wheeler on my own. Like any normal person, I wanted a motorcycle and a jet on day one, but this was far better than the minefields of Catch-22s I had faced in California. As I grew within the field and got my medical life back on track, the company began paying me more. I wished it had been faster, but again, even my salary had training wheels.

When I first met my boss, he said, "Let me get this straight. I'm going to hire you as an intake coordinator. Eventually you'll be treating patients. After that, once you've picked my brain and learned everything I know, you'll leave me and become my competition. Am I right?" Was this a trick question? On another day in a different year I would have obfuscated, if not lied straight out, but I'd been through a lot and done a lot of lying and most of it had not served me well, so I tried the truth. "Yeah, sure, that sounds like a great plan!" He laughed, I laughed, and a good time was had by all. But at the core, humor is usually a big peach pit of truth. Truth was, we both knew that really was the master plan, whether I knew it or he approved of it or not. Only a completely unambitious doctor would come to such a situation and think differently, and I had always been ambitious in my own way.

A nearby methadone clinic had a part-time opening I felt I could squeeze into my weekly schedule. I didn't know as much as I wanted to know about methadone, so I took the job—both for money as well as for educational advancement. Pretty soon I was making more at the methadone clinic than at my full-time job. Put the two salaries together, and while I was killing myself with the young-man's hours I was pulling, they started to add up and help Maurine and me get back up on our feet again.

Out of the blue I got a call from a doctor from the Rhode Island Medical Board. He had led the way in treating me decently and fairly, so I was happy to hear his voice on the other end of the line. He said to me, "Skip, I really admire your story and how you've cleaned up your act. You're a good guy. I have some clinics in Massachusetts. Would you like to start your own substance-abuse practice in one of my places?" I was dumbstruck. An angel had come to my rescue again. In spite of that, we couldn't quite come to terms. He wanted me to have a general practice as well and I not only felt somewhat disinterested in that; I considered myself ill-equipped to do such work at the same level of quality I was now doing the addiction work. A month went by and he reapproached me. What about an addiction-only practice in Rhode Island? Perfect.

He invested money in creating the practice and together we went to the bank and took out some loans. A short time later, Medical Assisted Recovery in Warwick, Rhode Island was born, and it is still my practice today. I was finally back.

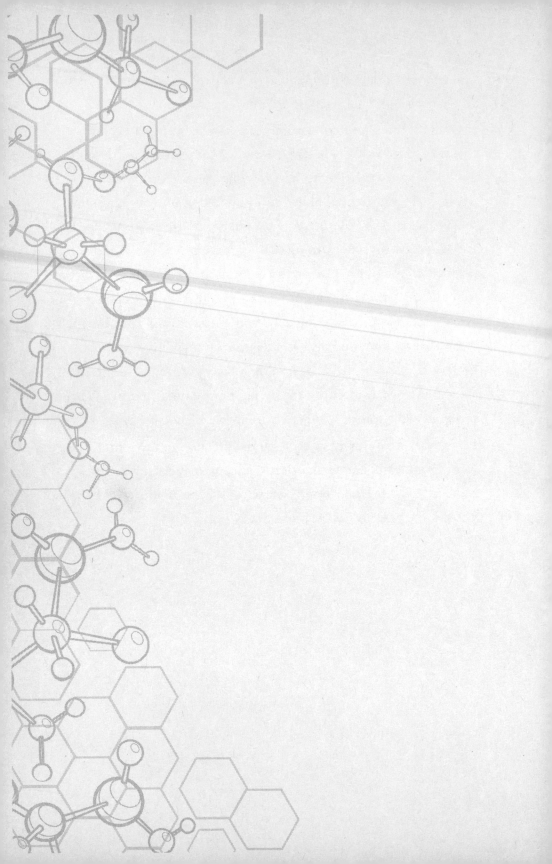

Rx

CHAPTER ELEVEN

THE REBIRTH OF DR. SKIP

Once I got my license back and immersed myself in the field of addiction medicine, I met a slew of wonderful practitioners and professionals. We started slowly. I set my sights on getting a nursing board contract. I suggested to the board I could develop an action plan for dealing with nurses who had drifted into addiction but wanted to get their lives back and return to work in nursing if they were able to attain and maintain recovery. We got the contract and it started a steady flow of nurses to my new practice.

My word is my bond with my patients. I am very strict. I'm
sometimes impatient with the lying that often accompanies
addiction because as a recovering addict, I know a lie when I
hear one. I know, because they try to use the same lies I used. I
feel an obligation to these patients. During my own recovery I
had a visceral reaction, a shudder of appreciation for the fact my
addiction never killed or harmed a patient. It's the sort of thing you
don't think about much at the time, particularly if you're impaired
whenever you're not wearing your white coat. But in recovery,
it plagued me, even though I had everything in the world to be
thankful for since nothing bad had ever happened as I practiced.
I'd been lucky, nothing more. But you can't bank on luck. Sober
doctors and nurses kill people, too. I vowed when dealing with other
medical practitioners I would treat them professionally, but not cut
them any slack. They had to understand the far greater weight that
rests on their shoulders, the danger they pose to innocent people.
The thought that I could look the other way while other medical
practitioners under my care compromised the health and safety
of their patients now scares me as much as my own professional
performance. It is two degrees of responsibility and I feel it acutely.

I developed a relationship with a urine drug-screening company
that has a system that allows me to test for just about every drug
commonly and uncommonly used by nurses and doctors. Medical
professionals can get their hands on things most street users don't
even know about or understand how to exploit for recreational
use—Ritalin and Fentanyl, for example—that most tox screens
don't even test for. I needed to be able to catch not just the usual
players like alcohol, heroin, and cocaine. I had to go after the sly
foxes of the prescription-drug trade.

I became certified as a medical review officer, which allows me to test, evaluate, and treat pilots, truckers, air traffic controllers, and such. Along with that I learned even more about drug testing. Ask people on the International Olympic Committee; it's like chasing a moving target. No sooner is a test developed to sniff out an offending drug, then some other methodology comes along to mask it. In my case, it's not that the kinds of patients I see are using sophisticated methods of masking; they're just finding newer and more creative ways to get high, ways we never thought to test for before.

Once my business partner chose to leave his seat on the Rhode Island Medical Board, we no longer had any conflicts of interest when it came to treating Rhode Island physicians. Thus began a second source of industry-specific patients. We also began to treat pharmacists, paramedics, and lawyers. The "medical" in "Medical Assisted Recovery" is relatively new in this field. In the past, treatment of addiction has been primarily behavioral. The whole field is changing as rapidly as any other field of medicine.

We have an intensive outpatient group we hold three times a week, which we keep pretty full. It's for people who don't qualify for an inpatient program in which they leave home and stay in a facility for twenty-eight days. Some of these patients have just come out of a short-term detoxification at general hospitals, some after twenty-eight-day inpatient programs, and some are brand new to treatment. The group setting is every bit as important as our didactic approaches. It provides a supportive medium for treatment. What we talk about is great, but like other group programs, one of the most important takeaways is for addicts to see there are others just like them—that they are not alone nor are they or their stressors unique.

I'm sure this all sounds rosy and indeed it is. But just because you're experiencing recovery and turning your life around does not mean you're immune to life's potholes and tragedies, large and small. When bad things do happen, if you're aware, you're always checking yourself: *Is this going to make me start using again? Can I handle this crisis or will it send me reeling once more?*

My first major pothole came from the fact I'd never really handled my own billing. Odd, I know, but when I was an ER doc, I either drew a salary or I was a contract employee or contractor. Never did I personally have to navigate the utterly confusing morass that is the health insurance system in America. I got paid by the hospital. But in my new practice, I got tons of provider forms to fill out, and I answered every question honestly. I chose not to apply for a Medicare or Medicaid number because our practice was not going in that direction. When I filled out provider forms for other insurance companies, if they asked for those numbers, I clearly stated I did not have them and I did not participate. What I did not know is you need those numbers for practically everything—but no one told me that from the outset. Meanwhile, we were up and running, seeing patients, submitting bills, and being paid by insurance companies. Our little locomotive was chugging along just fine.

About a year into the practice, I got a certified letter from a major insurance provider, our biggest source of income, stating I had committed fraud. Fraud? Somehow, it all came back to the issue of not having a Medicare or Medicaid number—which I told them we did not have nor did we desire to have the day I applied to be one of their participating doctors, and they accepted me anyway. They said they were dropping me as a provider and asked me to refund them every penny they had ever paid us. No due process, no hearing, no appeal, but suddenly I was expected to cough up a significant portion of our first year's revenue, *plus* I was being called a fraud.

I was despondent. I had filled out all the forms truthfully, yet they used the term "fraud," which was a massive punch to the gut. My old shame reared its ugly head. I had to go outside and take a deep breath. They were trying to put me down on the mat again, only this time I wasn't going to let them. I was going to fight this. In California, I'd been in the wrong. I screwed up. But this time I'd done nothing wrong. Instead of letting it get to me, I was going to convert all my stress and depression into positive action.

I was referred to the sharpest and nicest attorney I had ever met, who fought like mad for me. It took a lot of time—insurance companies make their money by denying coverage, denying payment, and winning wars of attrition. But in the end, we won our appeal. The settlement was that we did not have to repay *all* the money they'd paid us—they insisted on saving face by penalizing us somewhat—and we could go back to business taking their insurance and seeing their patients. This still left us owing legal fees as well, which our attorney rightly deserved. We'd also lost a lot of money by having turned away some patients. A few weeks later, a smaller insurance company came along and pulled the exact same stunt with us. Once more, I went to our lawyer. Once more she helped us win. Once more, despite winning, I had to pay for her services and we still had to pay a settlement fee or else spend even more money beating the insurance carrier in court. This is one reason Americans hate health insurance companies.

It was finally over and I'd been vindicated. It was still a major setback for a new practice, though. It also galled me that here I was, someone people were willing to take a risk on and give a second chance, and now something came along again to put a shadow over my reputation. It makes you a little crazy, like you want to grab every stranger you see on the street and say, "You don't know me, but I'm a good guy. Skip Sviokla. If you ever hear that name and someone says something bad about me, that's all in the past. I've been good. I'm a decent guy." They call it the wreckage of the past. It follows you so any new problems that come into your life somehow get connected to those bad old days, even if it's only in your own head. I worried about the rumor mill. Would referring doctors hear about this new "scandal" and think, "Oh yeah, isn't that guy the drug addict? Yeah, he's probably guilty of something."

Luckily, the Rhode Island Medical Society, which had helped direct and oversee my addiction recovery, had a good impression of me since many people there came to know me on a more personal basis as time went by, and got to look past my "rap sheet" and see the real me. They asked me to speak at local physicians' groups and hospitals to talk about the dangers of addiction within the medical community. Eventually, I began giving annual talks to the incoming house staff at Rhode Island Hospital, the largest acute care center in the state. The talks were and are still well-received. Fifteen percent of all medical professionals have addiction problems, but the good news is they tend to have the best recovery statistics. Why? The same reason I'm alive today: if we hit bottom, we have nowhere to go but up . . . or into the ground. Our occupations are more stringent than most, less forgiving. We carry a big, pink neon sign around our necks, like an ex-con, when we are forced to try to find work in another field. We're almost unemployable, which I learned the hard way. That's a heck of a motivation toward recovery. Medical boards also insist on a lot of enforced monitoring and treatment before they allow us to return to the field of treatment, which is a recipe for success. I tell addicted doctors that the sooner they seek help, the better.

I also direct my comments to the other 85 percent, the majority who are not and will never become addicts. I tell them, "Listen and learn. Study your patients well. Addicts are great liars. How else did I get to the age of fifty before anyone found out I was an addict? The presence of addiction is a complicating factor in most any assessment or treatment of any malady. Addicts are not just homeless people muttering to themselves, pushing a shopping cart down the street. I was a high-flying doctor with country club memberships and luxury cars. Yet I was every bit as addicted as the bum in the gutter. If you are giving your patients good treatment yet something remains wrong, consider the possibility your patients may be addicts. Most will deny it and most of the time you will be relieved to hear that, because most doctors don't want to deal with addicts; it's not why you went into medicine. You've taken an oath to respect life and you've probably come to view addicts as people who do not respect life— —theirs or the lives of the people they may injure through their actions while impaired. But treat them you must."

I even provide an elective course in addiction medicine for internal medicine residents. Frankly, I wish it were a mandatory course not just for personal reasons, but because of how important knowledge in this field is to medical professionals. Addiction is so commonplace in our world. It's not that I feel we need so many more physicians specializing in the field, but even if you want to be an internist, a surgeon, or a urologist, I guarantee you will have dealings with addicts, who you may or may not recognize as such. But still, things are far better now than when I was a medical student. Back then, we had literally nothing. No one came in and discussed drug abuse with us. We were never asked to face down the possibility we may already be or may someday become addicts. As this educational movement continues in the training of physicians and nurses, it will become far less likely anyone will have to go through the experience I had in California.

I believe in rehabilitation. Unless you plan on giving someone the electric chair, you have to deal with the fact he or she will someday be out in society, and we'd all better plan for it. Making an example of me the way they did was punishment without real thought of rehabilitation. Humbly speaking, had I not moved, the course that was laid out would not only have been a loss to me and my family, it would have been a loss to society as well, considering the many patients and medical professionals whose lives I've affected since my recovery. Medical boards are slowly reaching out for more treatment versus more punishment, and nursing boards are always looking to create more awareness, since nurses are so exposed to opioids and other prescription medications.

It shouldn't surprise you if you think about it, that nurses fall prey to prescription drug addiction more often than doctors. The next time you're in a hospital, see who handles the drugs. It's never doctors. Doctors write out a prescription on a piece of paper and hand it to a nurse and the nurse fills it. The nurse goes to the hospital pharmacy or the automated dispensing machine and gets the pills and hands them to the patient. In the simplest form of abuse, all the nurse has to do is not give the patient the pill and claim she did. Most patients are so out of it they have no idea what they should be given and when. And how would they know if they were slipped a placebo? If a patient is supposed to get six painkillers in a twenty-four-hour period and only gets four, who is the wiser? If the patient complains of lack of pain relief, the doctor ups the prescription to a more frequent or larger dosage or stronger meds, and the nurse continues on with the deception. It's a nifty set-up for an addict.

Medical professionals, because they have so much to lose, tend to be the least-forthcoming patients when it comes to admitting their addiction or substance abuse. They are likely to dig in harder and rail against the label "addict" even when they are caught red-handed. I have other patients—blue- and white-collar workers in other fields—who either get it right away or they don't, but a far higher percentage of them either walk into my office admitting their problem right off the bat, or come to admit it fairly early on in treatment. I think a lot of it is because medical professionals continue to save lives even while addicted. They tend to rationalize more than the average person. "I worked a twelve-hour shift and saw thirty-two patients. Perhaps I take some pills now and then (usually *a lot* of pills), but I hold it together so . . . no problem." When caught, they're forced to admit they took pills, but deny it's a problem. I even coined a phrase for my nurse-patients: deRNial. Some nervously chuckle when I write it on a whiteboard, with the big "RN" in the middle of the word. Others get upset. Nurses often harbor a lot of well-deserved defensiveness about their profession. They are incredibly well-educated and well-trained, they take a lot of crap from doctors and patients, and despite their vast training, long hours, and hard work, they are incredibly underpaid. If that's not temptation to want to dull the pain of reality, I don't know what is. I did, though, have one quick-witted nurse see my invented word on the board and rebut with, "Yeah, well we think 'MD' stands for 'Malignant Denial.'" Touché.

In the midst of running my new practice, my knee got so arthritic I needed a total joint replacement. This is always an area of concern for someone who once abused opioids: how do you deal with the major pain of surgery that literally mandates your physician prescribe painkillers for you? I could get hooked again.

I arranged to have a regimented inpatient detox from the drugs they had to put into my system during the actual operation. I could not allow that stuff to stay in my body any longer than absolutely necessary. It is also typical to start receiving oral opioids hours after the operation. At the last minute, I had a change of heart and told the doctor to skip that step. Good idea, I thought. Not so good, I found out. When I awoke and they removed my IV about twelve hours after surgery, I began physical therapy with nothing but Tylenol in my system. That was stupid. The pain was excruciating. I wouldn't wish it on the Yale football team. A machine keeps moving your knee up and down, and with each movement I bit down so hard I thought I'd crack my teeth. Meanwhile, they put me in the cardiac ward rather than the orthopedic ward. Cardiac nurses aren't used to ortho patients and their unique needs, and in general, nurses hate when doctors are patients. We're pain-in-the-ass know-it-alls, which nobody likes. I had to beg those nurses for my Tylenol, which an ortho nurse would have had at the ready. But in the end, I got through the entire process without a single oral opioid touching my tongue. I felt like the veteran of a war. I would never advise a patient of mine to be that hardcore about the whole experience. It was unnecessary zeal on my part.

Recovery has other areas where overzealousness can be a hazard. We're told to avoid people who do not respect our recovery and tempt us to fall off the wagon. Some recovery groups take this

a little too far and become almost cult-like in their isolationism.
The middle ground for me is I've had very few people I've had
to cut out of my life. Looking back, I never had a ton of real, true
friends—just acquaintances, and acquaintances come and go. If my
sole activity with them was going out and pounding down some
drinks, those acquaintances no longer had use for me and vice-
versa. If friends and acquaintances are willing to listen, I tell them
abstinence is the only answer for an addict; there are no vacations
from recovery. If they understand, great; if they don't, good-bye.
For an addict, the stove is always hot and if you touch it, even for
a moment, you get burned. Moving all the way across the nation
helped. It helps other addicts, too, if they can afford it. Most of the
people I used with, I left behind in California. Back east, I rejoined
the Harvard Club in Boston and I go there with Maurine and the
kids. I love showing off the place to my grandchildren and planting
seeds in their heads about someday matriculating at that marvelous
school in Cambridge and having their own membership at the old
Back Bay Club. Decades ago, I drank every time I visited the place.
Today I abstain. I don't miss that at all.

   With my family and extended family, things are pretty good. I
have one relative who uses too heavily for my taste and we had to
part ways. I got into recovery before my 106-year-old grandmother
died, which made both of us really happy. As for my children,
they've all been fantastic. With four kids, you would think there'd
be a variety of reactions and attitudes, but they've all been very
forgiving. They all have different personalities, but not one of them
took longer to warm to me than the others. I felt the worst about
Chip, as he was the youngest as well as the only boy. By the time I
was at my lowest, the girls were all living on their own, even though

I occasionally invaded their space when I had nowhere else to go due to my own bad behavior. But they were older and more mature by then. Chip needed things from me I was unable to give him, things I'd been able to give the girls when they were the same age— not just monetary things, but emotional support and advice. Who wants advice from a drunk? And whereas high school and college-age girls naturally gravitate to their mother for certain things, where was I for my only son? I apologize to him perhaps the most, but he's incredibly good about it and always stops me in my tracks. At times I wonder if all my kids are in denial and someday they're going to open up and tell me what horrible things I had done to them, but so far it hasn't happened.

When I visit Nicole in Rye, New York, she brings me to some private clubs to which she belongs. She introduces me to her friends like I'm some kind of hero, which is a strange way to look at my life, if you're asking me. But maybe that's how she's coping with it. To hear her tell it, I overcame this incredible thing, like I survived an avalanche or ran some race on two artificial legs. On my return visits, everyone seems to remember me. It's an odd feeling, since in my prior life I felt I had to buy lots of drinks and give big tips to get that same level of respect. My, how things have changed, and how very much I've learned. Nicole has always had my back.

My kids drink. I don't really mind, although I watch them carefully. It would kill me if I passed my disease along to them genetically or environmentally. So far, though, so good. I never see them drink to numb the blues, which is a good sign. But I'm watching; I'm watching. Maurine, of course, *never* fails to help me keep things in perspective. I love her for standing by me and I owe her everything. Without her I couldn't have made it.

R_X
EPILOGUE

There are a lot of addicts out there. Some may see themselves
in my story, while others may know friends or family members
who mimic my personal profile. I am living proof addiction can
happen to anyone, not just to the usual suspects. Furthermore,
we are no longer living in a society where addiction is limited to
alcohol, heroin, cocaine, and similar "party drugs" or street drugs.
Prescription medicine addiction and abuse is probably the fastest-
growing area of addiction since we, as a society, are surrounded by
the stuff. It has exceeded the popularity of heroin. Some folks are
getting addicted when they are doing little more than trying to find
legitimate medical relief from pain and suffering.

Hypochondria is often a gateway to addiction. Where once we felt **pain,** now we know we can go and get pain relief. This should be hailed as a medical marvel, and it is, but it becomes a matter of method, degree, and perception. Life is full of aches and pains, but knowing a pill can make them all go away, some of us take the plunge into oral opioid overkill. Pretty soon patients begin to take opioids prophylactically—as a preventative measure. Then there is the problem of the body developing a tolerance to oral opioids. Maybe we really are in pain—or else we've convinced ourselves that phantom pain is real—and we need ten tabs of Vicodin to get relief where one used to do it. When a doctor tries to cut us off or cut us down, we "doctor shop," which thank God is becoming harder and harder to do with the dawning of electronic medical records but still, it happens. Eventually, some people become hooked and start mimicking the behaviors of addicts who use street and party drugs—going to shady characters and paying any amount of money just to get relief. These addicts are sometimes difficult to reach because they are convinced addicts behave in a far different manner than they do. They've bought into the stereotype of the guy who wakes up every day to a tumbler of rum, or the junkie who shoots heroin in a gritty flophouse with a communal needle. What isn't realized is that it doesn't matter how you get there, it's that the end point is the same—you're an addict. If you stop, you'll feel sick and in hellacious pain, and so you dose and dose and dose.

Awareness. Discipline. These are words easier said than done, but it begins by keeping an honest and open line of communication going with your physician. Trust him or her with the truth. There are non-narcotic interventions for chronic pain—massage, heat or cold, electro-stim, biofeedback, epidural, and surgery. Medicating away pain has become a chronic problem in this country, and it can be avoided. It also takes forward-thinking doctors. Decades ago, there were more lazy practitioners who found it easier to hand out opioid scripts like candy. I see that changing, but it's not quite there yet. Furthermore, it requires more than the simple step of refusing to fill more prescriptions for an overusing patient. The doctor may have unknowingly created an addiction in that patient. This means he or she has a responsibility to treat that patient as one would an addict. The patient *is* now an addict. The patient should be brought down off their addiction by a medical specialist trained in doing so. Cold turkey is not only painful and cruel, if often fails because the patient left writhing alone on the floor is liable to do some very desperate things in order to get relief. Withdrawal should be medically monitored, and practices like mine offer that service, as do many others. I envision a day when oral opioids will no longer be given for the treatment of pain at all, and it will be a good move because over long periods of time— even moderate periods of use—it simply does not work. Besides, pain is not a diagnosis, it is a symptom. If you break your arm, I could give you opioids for the pain, but your arm would still be broken. For as much as no doctor would ever treat a broken bone that way, we must look at all pain in a similar fashion—what is the root cause of the pain, and how can we address it in the long term?

Amphetamines. A problem that appears on the wane, yet still exists in certain geographic pockets, is over-diagnosis of attention deficit/hyperactivity disorder (ADHD) treated with various forms of amphetamines. Some schools have a policy of ridding their classes of misbehaving students by suggesting to parents that medical intervention is required for their sons or daughters to reenter the classroom. Simply interpreted, this means, "Either put your kid on Ritalin (a form of 'speed') or he or she will be expelled." Like opioids, amphetamines can be addictive and in the aforementioned situation, we are turning kids into speed addicts when many of them do not even suffer from acute ADHD. We also have high-achieving students, some under pressure to perform well at top high schools and colleges, faking symptoms in order to be misdiagnosed with ADHD, or else buying it illegally on the street, in order to work longer and harder and do better on tests and papers. Even the kid who downs ten energy drinks and ten espressos to pull an all-nighter is committing a form of drug abuse. And drug abuse can easily lead to drug addiction. Worse yet, many of these amphetamines are not picked up by standard drug testing methods, and users are even more apt to deny they are addicted. Again, the kid misdiagnosed with ADHD, or the high-achiever trying to stay competitive with his or her peers, does not match the cliché of the common street junkie. But if you find yourself or someone you love feeling the need to take amphetamines every day in order to function, you or that person may need a visit to an addiction-medicine specialist.

Is ADHD real? Yes. But I suggest before spending a cursory visit with a general practitioner and getting a script for Adderall or Ritalin, visit a good neuro specialist who will usually give hours and hours worth of testing before proclaiming a patient to have ADHD. Ironically, a study was recently done looking back on the mass of patients formerly diagnosed with ADHD and prescribed amphetamines. The ones who truly did have ADHD were actually the least likely to abuse the drugs. They only took them when necessary, which is as it should be.

Antidepressants. Luckily, drugs in the Prozac family (Zoloft, Paxil, etc.) are almost non-abuseable because, for one thing, most do not work right away. It takes weeks and weeks of steady use until the first sparks of efficacy appear. This is counterintuitive to a person with addictive tendencies. If I had to drink all day, every day, for six weeks before I could feel drunk, I would never have done it. On the other hand, there are some drugs lumped in with the term "antidepressant" by laypeople, that are really sedatives—Valium, Xanax, Klonopin, etc. These *are* more addictive. Tolerance can occur, and efficacy can be instantaneous.

There are people in this world suffering from real depression. Probably the simplest way of defining clinical depression is that a clinically depressed person is depressed regardless of whether there is anything to truly be depressed about. Example: a loved one dies. This is a naturally depressing thing that occurs in people's lives. To not be depressed about it would be unusual. To medicate ourselves when this occurs is wrongheaded, in my medical opinion, particularly if a fast-acting, potentially addictive sedative is prescribed. On the other hand, someone who spends all of their days *feeling* as if a loved one has died, or dreading that someday a loved one will die, is more likely suffering from real depression and should be seen by a medical professional who will likely treat them with a nonaddictive (or far less potentially addictive) SSRI such as Prozac or Celexa.

As a doctor, I see a lot of comingling of prescription medications, causing addiction. Patients go to Doctor A for depression, which they may or may not have, then Doctor B for pain relief, which they may or may not need, and they end up with some incredible problems. As doctors, we must take good histories and assume patients sometimes lie. We must study cases as thoroughly as possible and look to drug abuse as a possible answer to otherwise unanswerable questions in diagnosis. My highly intensive tox screens have turned up some crazy things—all sorts of prescription-drug combinations. Yes, some of these patients are knowingly abusing drugs, yet others are merely operating under the assumption that we live in a day and age when there is a pill for everything and if we take enough pills, everything in our lives will be rosy—no pain, no suffering, no unhappiness.

If you find yourself taking more and more prescription drugs, a big red flag should go up. Your doctor should notice it before you do, but if he or she does not, raise the issue yourself. Yes, in order to find the proper level for a particular drug to be effective in a certain patient, the doctor may have to start off small and scale up the dosage. But if a level of effectiveness is reached and it only stays there for a while until you feel the need to go up higher and higher, don't be afraid to ask questions. Go for a second opinion. And at all times, be honest with your caregivers. Tell them everything you are taking and be honest about your drinking and other activities (marijuana, cocaine, etc.). As a doctor, I knew what I was doing when I got addicted to opioids. I see far too many patients who get hooked and did *not* set out to abuse drugs. It crept up on them. This can be avoided by being proactive. It's one thing to have to take a daily dose of some medication because your thyroid does not function properly; it is a completely different situation when you feel the need for a sleeping pill each and every night. Get off the carousel and try nondrug interventions before you get addicted. More is not better. More means you're developing a problem. I recently treated a patient who was taking twenty sleeping pills a day, every day. That's addiction, my friend. By the time it gets that bad, you need an addiction specialist to bring you down safely. I don't say this to drum up business. Ask any ethical doctor. In a perfect world, we'd rather have *no* patients requiring our specialty. If you yell "Stop!" long before you reach the point of taking that much medication that often, you'll never need to see a doctor like me.

If you live in a large metropolitan area, finding second opinions and specialists shouldn't be a problem. If you live in a more remote region, try calling your state medical society if you need some ideas or referrals. Scour the Internet for addiction-medicine specialists in your area. The specialty is growing exponentially. But remember— an addiction specialist can help get you off of whatever you're addicted to, but if there remains an underlying medical problem— say you're addicted to painkillers because you have a bad back—we want you off the painkillers, but we also want you to not be in pain. I can't help you with your back, but another type of doctor can. Speak to your state medical society to find such a doctor, one who will try different approaches rather than just tossing potentially addictive meds at you.

Because things move so quickly, by the time this book is in your hands there may be even newer concepts in the marketplace of ideas for the treatment of addiction. Innovation is the key to achieving greater degrees of success. One thing we are doing now at my practice is "motivational interviewing." Gone are the days when we first felt the need to "break down" addicts—get them to bottom out and admit addiction in order to seek help. Now, we feel it is an important first step to simply get them talking to someone, anyone, but preferably someone educated in the field, in order to begin a dialogue with them about a possible addiction problem they may be experiencing. Instead of chastising or arguing with people, we try to listen and go to where they are on their personal journey and figure out what to do with them next. What is best for the patients and how do we get them there? It's an old saw to say you catch more bees with honey than with vinegar, yet we haven't always acted that way when it comes to addiction. Once you get people talking, you can assess if they are in "soft denial," "hard denial"; are they considering making a change but do not know how? Have they tried a few things but failed? The possibilities are endless. We go wrong when we treat any disease in cookie-cutter fashion, particularly one with a psychological component. With motivational interviewing, the goal is to make interviewees feel good that they reached out—positive reinforcement.

The two things I've learned from my addiction are realizing when there is a problem and understanding I can't control it. You'll see that sentiment in a lot of books and programs but I had to live it myself to understand its truth. I was always in denial, and I always felt I could simply reduce my intake and keep things at an acceptable level of non-impairment. I could not. If you can have one glass of wine every Friday night and no more, you are not an addict. If you cannot do that, or if you can only do that once in a while, while most other times downing sixteen shots of Scotch, you're an addict. You have a problem. Once I was able to spend time with recovering addicts who were happy—and that's the key word—*happy* not taking a drop of alcohol or a pill or a toot, I finally realized *I'm one of those people! Not only can I attain happiness this way, it is the only way for me to remain happy.*

Medically and scientifically, we are constantly trying to discover why Person A can be happy with one drink once in a while—can even drink to the point of impairment once a year perhaps—and someone like me could never fathom leaving half a glass of wine undrunk, even if it were glass number seventeen of the night. Surely there is a scientific answer to this. And yet there is not, at least not yet. We study the human genome and while we discover a difference between addicts and nonaddicts, there appears to be no single gene that is actionable, which we can change that will allow a person to go from being an addict to being a social drinker. Perhaps in the future there will be some sort of breakthrough in this area of science, but so far, those prospects look dim.

For some people, there is a greater or lesser effect from the release of dopamine when certain drugs are in the brain. Also, some people don't break down their alcohol as fast and become sick after only a drink or two. Unfortunately, this does not mean they have a natural rejection of addiction, since this phenomenon is limited only to alcohol and they can get addicted to other things just as easily as the next person. Bottom line: sans a biological imperative where we can treat a genetic disorder to prevent or stop addiction, the main difference between a person with a problem and one without is whether one feels a strong desire to be truly impaired and why. I drank and did drugs to escape. When two people go to a party and use too much, one can be an addict while the other is not based strongly upon that big question: *why?* The addict wanted to escape something, while the other person may have simply gotten lost or distracted in the moment, felt bad about it the next day, vowed not to do it again (at least in the immediate future), and likely kept that promise for a reasonable length of time without feeling significant temptation. The addict wakes up miserable and begins looking for chemically-based ways of feeling less miserable, maybe even happy, for a short while. When my life was at its worst, I drank and drugged to escape. Maurine is a social drinker. Never during those dark days did she increase her drinking one iota. Never did she look at our turmoil and say, "Boy, I need a drink." That's what makes me an addict while she is not.

Beware the morning drink or morning drug. If you feel the need to counterbalance the withdrawal symptoms of the night before—the "hair of the dog" theory—you've got a problem. If you grimace at the thought of facing another day on this earth sober when you haven't even had a chance for anything bad to happen yet—you've got a problem. And if you've got a problem, get help. Help is always only a phone call away.

True recovery is not simply about giving up substance use. Abuse must be replaced with something else, a more positive force in one's life. If the only change you make is to stop using, there's a great likelihood you'll fall off the wagon someday. Instead, find other outlets. Pursue your bliss. Create relationships. Only then will you stop hanging onto recovery with white knuckles, like it's a speeding roller coaster with no safety harness.

I really think neuro-imaging may eventually lead us to new innovations in the understanding and treatment of addiction. Functional MRIs are helping physicians see and thus treat problems such as severe OCD, either with invasive brain procedures using lasers, or even newer methods, using directed magnetic fields. There are things going on in the brain we still do not fully understand when it comes to why some people become addicts while others manage to avoid it. It's not limited to seeing what happens to the pleasure centers when an addict is sated. I believe it is equally interesting to discover—if we can—what happens in the brain when an addict finally "gets it," when he or she surrenders to the power of the illness. I compare it to the artwork of M.C. Escher, the guy who draws all those works where you can't really tell if the stairs are going up or coming down, whether there are dark birds on a white background or white birds on a dark background. The basics of substance abuse are well-known. It's like smoking. There is no human being alive today who does not know smoking is bad for you. Yet smokers still smoke. But then one day, some quit. Why? We know it's not because there was some truly new information presented to them. The same goes for drug and alcohol addiction. Why do recovering addicts have that "moment of clarity"? The more spiritual among us claim it is the Higher Power. I am a man of science. I demand to understand scientifically how that works. To this very day I cannot explain to you what changed for me the day I was up on the roof above the yoga studio and said, "Okay, I'm done. No more drinking and drugging." I'd like to know that, and if I could ever discover what change went on in my brain that day, it might give us an insight into better ways of medically treating addiction. There is not a single thing I knew the day before my moment of clarity I did not know the day after it. So why the disconnect between knowing, and acting upon that knowledge?

A large portion of my practice is people from regulated professions, such as doctors, nurses, and lawyers. When I had my troubles in California, I was punished and cut loose. Today, in Rhode Island and other forward-thinking states, when a professional is caught using as I was, he or she is indeed punished, but instead of being cut loose he or she is instead immediately placed into a program if he or she desires to ever return to that profession. That's a great thing. As a participant in this program, I understand the moment a person is caught using, he or she is not necessarily fully ready to recover, but it's a great time to move in that direction. Indeed, I have some professionals who will likely never get their licenses back. They may die while still in denial, or simply feel they enjoy being high more than they like working in their field. Nonetheless, I wish I'd been put into a monitored program when I was caught. I doubt I would have suffered as badly and put my family through as much as I did. This system is far better. We don't move the goalposts capriciously. If a person takes the well-laid-out steps put before him or her, and if he or she complies with compulsory treatment and monitoring, passing his or her random urine tests, then he or she will eventually be able to return to his or her field. That's fair, and in life, all we ask is fairness. It's the difference between being treated like a patient with an illness versus being treated like a criminal. Even criminals have probation programs and halfway houses—access to schooling and training while incarcerated. I was tossed out like the trash. I don't say that in hopes of eliciting sympathy; I say it because it's a poor system. Treatment works. People can be rehabilitated.

Addiction is a medical problem *but* . . . I cannot diminish the need to take personal responsibility. There are boots solidly planted in both camps, each saying it is one or the other. I believe it is primarily medical, but personal responsibility does indeed play a role.

Families of addicts also need to help where they can. The addict must be assumed guilty until proven innocent. Addicts always claim to not be impaired. If they appear impaired, they are impaired.

Families must confront such behavior as early and often as possible, in a loving and supportive way. Yelling at an addict will not bring about change, but neither will ignoring his or her addiction. Be honest with the addict and support his or her efforts toward recovery. Do not enable.

I believe I am alive today because of my loving family. This does not mean they were soft on me. Maurine never enabled me. She did not leave me, but she certainly was never in denial about me. She gave me tough love. We make a pledge of "for better or for worse, in sickness and in health." Lots of people want to marry a doctor. But how many would stay with that doctor when he'd lost it all and appeared to have no chance of ever getting any of it back—an incorrigible addict?

I also benefited by moving away from where I'd displayed my most addictive tendencies. A change of scenery is very helpful when seeking recovery. If you can do that, do it. It gets you away from those you used with and away from your sense-memory triggers— the old bar you used to frequent, the business that fired you, etc.

As a young man, I made it to Harvard. That wasn't easy. I fell from Harvard to hell. I'm sure I'm not the first to do that. But looking back on my life, it's the "and back" part I'm most proud of. There were times I doubted I'd ever be a respectable member of society again, let alone a doctor. And today I live with a renewed vigor and passion for life I haven't felt since I was an aspiring young surgeon. I didn't just come back to medicine; I filled my life with happiness, satisfaction, and accomplishment that only comes from doing good works that fill the soul. I don't think I will ever use again. Why should I? Life doesn't get any better than this.

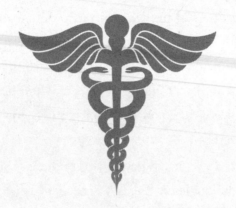